CRM

W9-CMR-100

Moonlight Sonata at the Mayo Clinic

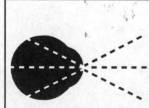

This Large Print Book carries the Seal of Approval of N.A.V.H.

MOONLIGHT SONATA AT THE MAYO CLINIC

NORA GALLAGHER

THORNDIKE PRESS
A part of Gale, Cengage Learning

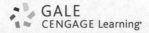

GALE
CENGAGE Learning·

Detroit • New York • San Francisco • New Haven, Conn • Waterville, Maine • London

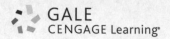
GALE
CENGAGE Learning®

LIBRARY OF CONGRESS CATALOGING-IN-PUBLICATION DATA

Gallagher, Nora, 1949–
    Moonlight sonata at the Mayo Clinic / by Nora Gallagher. — Large print edition.
        pages cm — (Thorndike Press large print health, home & learning)
    ISBN 978-1-4104-6324-1 (hardcover) — ISBN 1-4104-6324-9 (hardcover)
    1. Gallagher, Nora, 1949– —Health. 2. Sarcoidosis—Patients—Biography. 3. Uveitis—Miscellanea. 4. Large type books. I. Title.
    RC182.S14G35 2013b
    616.4'29—dc23   2013025963

Published in 2013 by arrangement with Alfred A. Knopf, Inc., a division of Random House, Inc.

Printed in the United States of America
1 2 3 4 5 6 7 17 16 15 14 13

For the good doctors: Babji Mesipam, Doreen Burks, Robert Wright, Narsing Rao, Clarke Stevens, and Robert Baughman; and for physician's assistant, William P. Holland

About suffering they were never wrong,
The Old Masters: how well they understood
. . . how it takes place
While someone else is eating or opening a
   window
or just walking
dully along.

—W. H. Auden,
"Musée des Beaux Arts"

■ ■ ■ ■

PART ONE:
DROWNING

■ ■ ■ ■

CHAPTER 1

The year I drowned, I took the No. 6 train uptown in New York to the Hispanic Society of America to visit their collection of ancient maps. Among them are large maps, drawn by men who were claiming the new world not only for Spain but for Christianity. One had a crucifix at the top, and another was adorned with a Madonna. Still another had a Muslim soldier with a sword on one side of a map of Africa and an armed European on the other.

The pride of the museum was Juan Vespucci's map of the world, *mappa mundi*, completed in 1526. They keep it in a private room available only to scholars who sign up well in advance. I knocked on the door without much hope, but the thin, polite man who opened it said, "Of course," and let me in. Crowded into a small space were a number of wooden desks with a few people working at them, who looked up, then went back to their books and papers. On one whole wall was an old gold curtain with tasseled fringe, like something you would find in a drawing room. The man drew it back, and there it was: all that was known of the world. Africa very much in place; South America a crooked, narrow knee; North America only a scrap of land, surrounded by watery blurs where all knowledge ran out.

I was directed upstairs to an exhibit of smaller maps, laid out in glass cases in two darkened rooms. These maps were specific, precise, and individual, drawn by the pilots of ships, "to preserve," as the curator put it, "the Mediterranean sailors' firsthand experience of their own sea."

They were so carefully and beautifully decorated — castles with flags marked cities, compass roses and fleurs-de-lis were drawn along the edges — they may not have been working charts to be kept on board but beautiful replications of where the sailors had been and what they had seen, what the curator called "subjective truth."

Among the maps were practical books and charts called *derroteros* (in English, "courses" or "pathways") made by rutters or coastal pilots. These guides, with their close focus, aided mariners who plied both local and more international waterways and provided a bird's-eye view of shoreline elevations. The journals accompanying the maps had notes on the stars and entries regarding harbors and ports. One particular *derrotero* was displayed with its original hand-stitched hemp case. It was a painstaking map of a shoreline, with hundreds of tiny inscriptions and notes and small perfect houses drawn along the water's edge. Only by reading back and forth between different maps was a sailor able to orient himself.

I walked among these maps, often the only person in the dark rooms. And I began to see that I was navigating between the larger *mappa mundi* of organized religion and philosophies — Christianity, Buddhism, Judaism, Islam, and not to ignore, the Church of Atheism — big cosmologies with so much history and tradition, and so many power struggles behind them. Firm ideas. Fixed points. And my own *derrotero,* my firsthand experience of my own sea, my own subjective truth.

What principally drove the makers of the large maps was conquest; the smaller ones, discovery. My *derrotero* would be of the smaller coastline, the individual rock. I would draw it to tell others what to watch out for, what I learned. Or what I knitted together, what sufficed. No Essential Truth, but a geography worth recording.

We know from the work of biochemists that the very material from which life arose was dust blown here from some distant star that we will never see. That the carbon dioxide atoms that surround us today may have been breathed out by a woman or a man who lived here hundreds of years ago. That the world is made of shapes and materials that move and change, things we cannot know exactly but can often only apprehend.

Our desire to apprehend this world is often couched as a passive state, as *Belief,* a dumb acceptance. And sometimes I suppose it is. But the struggle to grasp what lies just outside our firm knowledge is in fact energetic. Reason runs out, and we reach beyond it, toward the blur at the edge of the map. And beyond that, toward what cannot be known. And this urgent need to reach beyond ourselves is not "real" until it has been worked through a human life, in its specificity, its particulars. Our lives, our bodies, are its mediums. Whatever the reality of this thing beyond us, the struggle toward it remains, oddly, individual. Like truth, what we sometimes call "faith" is alive. It changes. What drives us, as it drove

14

those sixteenth-century sailors, is discovery. Who knows in the end what we shall find out to be true; perhaps it's only what we ourselves held to honestly.

Like crossing a border
From one country to another in a second.

This is what I wrote down when I got home. I wrote it in a notebook and then added, *There will come a time in my life when the doctor says, "I am sorry. There is nothing I can do." I know this now, not in theory.*

It was an ordinary day. I had almost not gone to the doctor.

Dr. Lowe looked at my right eye. He said, "Darn." And I dropped out of the world I lived in, where I thought I knew about disease and vulnerability and death and *all that,* and entered another country. It was a spookily familiar world, same streets, same buildings, same people — a sci-fi version of my streets, my buildings, my people — but it was as if the furniture were slightly re-arranged, the people not quite right. It was not *like* another place; it *was* another country. It was like falling into Oz.

I walked right over the border without

knowing I was crossing it. It had no border patrol. I did no planning. I had no map. Dr. Lowe handed me the passport. I had it in my hands before I knew what it was. My ideas about illness and medicine and then "God" would soon be revealed for what they were: tickets on a train that had left the station.

The man Jesus had had quite a lot to say about losing. He was — now I understand — preoccupied with loss: lost sheep, lost coins, lost sons. His own lost life. The Hebrew scriptures emphasize exile. Islam: the stranger. The Buddhist Noble Truths: suffering. I had understood these sayings as metaphors. Not anymore.

In the end, I lost three things, and one of them was my faith.

I crossed Bath Street, parallel to Santa Barbara's hospital, and headed toward Castillo Street. I was careful to use the crosswalk. I felt the nearness of my own life, its centrality, its concreteness. Even then, early in my sojourn, in what I hoped was only a visit, not my destination, what was brought home to me was that I had taken my life for granted. A group of doctors in white coats was coming toward me, one eating a sandwich, another carrying a folder; a middle-

16

aged woman was talking on her cell phone — all of them just walking dully along as if their lives were not fragile. As if their lives were balloons . . . not a huge raft that had to be lugged along the sidewalk, a large body not possible to ignore because it . . . had . . . something . . . wrong . . . with . . . it. The raft is me. I am it. *They* are all walking around, nurses, doctors, visitors, on this block, and all over the world, as if their bodies were clothes or whatever, . . . They are — here is the right word — *oblivious.*

I had been there, not knowing that this was my creed, until ten minutes ago. The sick? Not me. The dying? Never. I had thought I knew. I'd had the flu. I'd had a cold. But these were not enough to dump me into Oz. Because I knew that eventually I'd get well. My time in the land of the sick had always been so short, it was like a layover. *I saw Thailand but only from the airport.* To pass into this place, you have to not know whether you are going to get out.

CHAPTER 2

In mid-November 2009, five months after seeing those maps in the museum in New York, I was building a fire in our house in Santa Barbara. Outside the weather was cold, but the winter rains had not yet begun. I had a queasy stomach, a fatigue so pronounced, I slept for three hours at a stretch, and I had a dull headache but no fever. I would repeat these symptoms in doctors' offices in Santa Barbara, in Los Angeles, and finally at the Mayo Clinic in Rochester, Minnesota. I had a queasy stomach. I had a headache. I was very, very tired. I would not say that I was building a fire — an important omission, as it turned out.

As I knelt on the hearth and leaned in to light the paper and pine kindling, I noticed a blur at the edge of my right eye, as if I had caught a ghost walking out of the room. Just at the periphery. This too I would repeat. "A blur," I would say, and the doctors or residents would lean toward me. "At the periphery."

I did not reach for the phone and call Dr. Lowe. I did not call him the next day. I didn't know, at that time, how quickly things can go wrong, how fast you can leave the ordinary world. I didn't know what a blur at the edge of the eye signifies.

I sat down in front of the fire and resumed reading *Wolf Hall* by Hilary Mantel, the last book, as it turned out, I would read for two years. The last book I have read, as I write these words.

My husband of twenty-seven years, Vincent, had left for New York, and I was to follow him in a few days. Both of us are writers, and New York for us, despite its expense, is our place: the world of writing and books and publishing, poetry readings, the dense concentration of friends who are artists and poets and novelists, shoptalk. The overheard conversations on the street. ("They told him, if he is a man, he has to be put in a man's cell.")

For six years we stayed in a studio in Greenwich Village owned by a friend who had moved to Maine, for a month at a stretch, three times a year. Our day jobs in California were part time. We wrote in the mornings — he in the entry hall, me in the

19

main part of the studio — before our colleagues on the West Coast woke up. Our friends charged us very little for what we got, but we still had to make extra money just to live in that city for a month (where, as a friend said, you might as well just throw dollar bills out the window). Vincent wrote catalog copy; I gave talks on my books and taught workshops.

In that nest we got to know how each neighborhood in New York is its own village. Around the corner from our building was a place called Typewriters and Things. The second time I went in there to buy a refillable pen, the Chinese American man who sold small black notebooks with lined pages and zippered lightweight mesh plastic bags in various sizes — for stray keys and whatever you needed to collect — that I have found nowhere else, remembered not only my name but our address in California. I went into our local shoe repair place — now extinct — and the Italian man who did not speak English sold me shoe trees for new boots. He took only cash, and when I said I didn't have any and turned to my husband, he said, *"È sempre così con le donne."* "It's always like that with women."

We went to New York for the rivers of words.

One of our goddaughters, who lived around the corner on Bank Street (with a roommate in a one-bedroom divided into two) while she went to NYU, dropped in one night and sat at our high table set in front of the windows. We drank glasses of pale wine and looked south at the Village, a historic district, much of it unchanged since the eighteenth century. Redbrick town-houses with aged vines splayed on a wall. Tarred rooftops. Chimneys shaped like pots. To the west, a watery flash, a sliver of the Hudson. And in the distance, the towers of Wall Street, like a chain of mountains.

"Let's do this forever," Carissa said.

But after the crash of October 2008, our friends who owned the apartment were forced to sell. We packed up the few things we had contributed — pots and pans, a computer screen, towels and sheets — and stored them in a friend's basement, hoping that we might someday find another place, then took the Long Island Rail Road to JFK. I cried all the way.

That November 2009 Vincent was to try out another apartment: a rent-controlled tenement (bathtub in the kitchen) on West 45th Street (where the friend who rented it was once awakened in the middle of the night by a man yelling, "Drug dealer in the building!" as if, she said, it were a public service announcement).

Part of me didn't want to go. I was reluctant to get on a plane, partly because I really felt sick. And partly because, I realize now, I had been traveling like a traveling fool, and I was worn out.

That year, 2009, I had left our house in California so many times I stopped counting. I packed the same suitcase with many of the same clothes. Printed out the boarding pass. Set the alarm. I was recognized as a business traveler. "When you walk in the door of the hotel room," a friend said, "ninety percent of the time, you don't have to look: the bathroom is on the right and the closet is on the left."

"Are you goin' out," a tall man from the South said to me as we entered a Boeing 737 together, "or comin' in?"

Miles piled up in my United account. I waited in line with the other Premiers, behind the 1 Ks and the Premier Executives, hoping for an upgrade. I lifted my bag into the overhead bin, nodded to the person sitting in the aisle seat, turned off my cell phone.

I traveled to Spokane, Sun Valley, Reno, San Francisco, New York, New Haven, D.C., Indianapolis, Austin. Into the business schedule, I packed family obligations. My former father-in-law, in Palo Alto, with whom I remained close, loved a visit. We have five godchildren with whom we like to check in. Vincent's father was very ill. Soon he would be dying.

My body was a machine that packed suitcases, lifted bags, printed out boarding passes. My mind knew where the bathroom and the closet would be while it worked on the next trip, the next talk, the next next. I was, as my godson Asa says, "bizzy."

In his poem "The Outpost," about being on patrol as part of his military service, Tomas Tranströmer, the Swedish Nobelist, tries to stay in the present, "to be where I am and to wait."

Instead, he finds, "things not yet happened" fill his thoughts.

Things not yet happened waited for me, at the periphery, crowding to get in.

I traveled like this to talk about my spiritual life, but the irony was lost on me. I have published two memoirs about faith and doubt, and a novel about a physicist's crisis of faith as he works on the atom bomb. My "religion" was neither certain nor fundamentalist (I was, after all, an Episcopalian), but I was a regular churchgoer. I had gone back to the Episcopal Church in my late

23

twenties, having joined it when I was thir-teen with my mother. She found an Episco-pal church in Albuquerque, St. John's Cathedral, with a priest who combined a passion for civil rights with fine liturgy. As a teenager, I fell in love with God and Father Kadey at the same time. One of my memo-ries of Kenneth Kadey — a stocky guy with a crew cut — was of him standing on a tall ladder in the middle of the church aisle changing a lightbulb in one of the huge chandeliers hanging from the cathedral ceil-ing, while talking to my mother about a civil rights protest.

My mother was what would be called now a "seeker." She had tried the First Congre-gational Church, when I was eight or nine, and must have gone to other churches in between then and the time we joined St. John's. I can't name what she was looking for, but I can guess. My parents' marriage took up a lot of space: my father, a lawyer, had been a drinking alcoholic; they sepa-rated for a year while we were living in Aspen. (Pretty towns were part of a search for happiness for her and new jobs for him.) Dad went back to Union Grove, Wisconsin, and lived on his sister's dairy farm that year. (My aunt wore tweeds, played chess by mail, and went to cattle shows in Denver.)

A man from AA sat with my dad through the night and day ahead while he suffered the DTs. A year later, after he had worked on an automobile assembly line in Kenosha to make money to bring back to us, my father came home, to Albuquerque, New Mexico, where we waited lined up — my mother, my brother, and I — for the stranger who got off the train.

We did not talk about God in my family. We talked about going to church and Father Kadey and marching for Dr. King. For a while I had a best friend who was a Roman Catholic, and I went to church with her because I liked the doughnuts her father bought for us on the way home. The Roman church service was pretty scary to me — the bleeding hearts, the fact that I could not take Holy Communion, the sins, the ringing of bells, the tapping of the heart — but I could see that the family organized itself around the church and belief. My family did not. I think for them it would have been impolite or vulgar.

When my father came home to us, he brought with him softball games, horses, an honest heart I could lean on, and AA. And his AA friends, who often gathered at our house and drank coffee and smoked cigarettes (I emptied the ashtrays into a silent butler), brought with them the thing they called Higher Power. They talked freely and openly about falling down drunk, about lying in the ditch, and about running out of any other option besides this Higher Power. If you had fallen off the edge, I understood finally, you could talk about God. Their stories were "grassroots religion," a friend said, and that's what it was.

I left off going to church when I was seventeen and went to college. I stayed away for ten years. I was working as a journalist in San Francisco then, stringing for *Time* magazine; my friends were artists and writers. I liked my work. I liked my friends. My life made sense but not enough sense. I found myself one Sunday in a beautiful dark-shingled church in the Marina District in San Francisco, crying.

My friends were leftists — some of them called themselves Marxists. They might have even read Marx. They had contempt for or fear of Christians. (Many of them were Jews, some of whom had been brought up to fear Christians.) So my decision to attend services at a pretty little church on Sundays was met with bafflement and condescension. "It looks like a hunting lodge," one writer said as he surveyed my church. My closest friend at the time wrote

26

me a long letter about how Christianity was nonsense.

But human beings require a larger story to fit themselves into. I was fitting my life into the larger story, the larger map, of Christianity.

I loved the liturgy of the Episcopal Church: the procession down the aisle, the cross held high, the kneeling at the communion rail. I loved the old words of the old prayers: "Almighty God, unto whom all hearts are open, all desires known, and from whom no secrets are hid."

I kept going to church, and I kept my religious views mostly to myself. When a woman in Berkeley complained that there were crucifixes on the walls of a Catholic high school where she had taken her daughter to visit as a prospective student, I did not say, What did you expect? I did not utter a word.

Later, married to Vincent and living in Santa Barbara, I worked in the soup kitchen housed in my church. I kept watch with dying friends. My brother, Kit, died of cancer in his fifties, much too young.

Finally I decided to write about my faith, my doubt, my struggle to understand these events. It was partly, I think, because of all those years of not speaking about it.

27

Now people wanted me to come and talk about what I had written. I was surprised and gratified when a church or a university invited me to give a talk or a reading (me?), so surprised that I always said yes.

I had become a religious professional without realizing it.

Gradually a crack between what I preached and what I practiced appeared and widened. I had the preaching part down, but the question was, what was my practice? Because of my travel schedule and the expectations placed on me, I lived in a state of anxiety. Before each and every speaking event, I felt terror, dread, and the desire to jump out of my skin. It started before leaving the house. I was not afraid of flying; somehow I gave up control once I got on the plane, but don't ask me to pack a bag and leave my living room.

I did not "pray." I did not have time. There was a lot of loss in my stories, but it was someone else's loss. I was in charge. I stood at podiums and pulpits, giving and giving, talking and talking, and meanwhile *the things not happened yet* occupied my mind like a colonial army. I might describe what was saving my life, but I did not know that something was killing me.

And there was a disconnect between what

I got from Sunday church and what, as it turned out, I needed. In the church service, there was a lot of "Almighty God." In the hymns, there was "A mighty fortress is our God." Yet in the gospels read each week, one heard about a man who knelt down and hugged children and said, "Be like them." Or who talked about lilies in the fields and swallows falling to the ground. This man healed someone every time he turned around: a blind beggar, a paralytic, a woman who couldn't stop menstruating. And all those lost things — the coins, the sheep, the son. This person — wasn't he the reason we were here? — seemed to have been relegated to the corners of the church, in the shadows, just outside our vision, on the periphery.

In "Suzanne," Leonard Cohen sings: "Jesus was a sailor when he walked upon the water and he spent a long time watching from his lonely wooden tower and when he knew for certain only drowning men could see him . . ." Only desperate men, I took this to mean. Only those who were lost.

I was, as it turned out, drowning, but my head was just enough above the water that I felt fine. I might be treading water with greater and greater speed, but you don't know you're drowning until you go under.

When I was not writing and speaking, I

worked for the environmental group within Patagonia, the outdoor clothing company. I am a part-time editor, the perfect day job for a writer. I write in the mornings and work for Patagonia in the afternoons. I have done this for over twenty years. Patagonia gives away one percent of sales to tough activists. At Patagonia too we did not always practice what we preached: one day one of our grantees came to visit us — this group of people hoping to help save steelhead trout and the Alaska wilderness and the river that ran right outside our doors, and she stood looking at us, with our heads bowed and our eyes glued to our computer screens. Finally she said, "Do you think maybe we could go outside?"

There is much to be said for the life I led. I was lucky. I loved seeing towns I'd never seen, on someone else's dime: I watched the Mississippi Falls one night in Minneapolis, woke to the mountains in Sun Valley, drank real bourbon in Louisville, drove late at night with a bunch of Episcopal priests to swing dance at the Broken Spoke outside Austin. I loved meeting people in Idaho and Indiana and Kentucky, places I might not have visited on my own. Where I went was based on a toss of a coin or a finger traced on a spinning globe.

In some of the parishes I visited, the idea of "small groups" was taking hold. In these gatherings, and the right climate, people were telling *stories*. I got to hear what people had found out about mystery or sacredness or what they called God, on the ground, in the trenches, outside of religious doctrine or within it, outside belief systems or within them. Inside churches, outside them. Once people had the freedom to talk about it, a wealth of knowledge emerged.

In a church in a suburban town in California, I met with the altar guild, all of them women, most of them elderly. They were the women who managed the practical side of communion: they washed the altar linens and then ironed them, kept track of the candles, ordered the wine and the wafers. Without them, the service would not happen.

One of them told me, with some embarrassment, that before putting the small cloths used to wipe the communion cup into the washing machine, she said a prayer that the stains would come out and the linens would get through the wash, and then that all the people in her church would get through, too.

At my own church, Trinity in Santa Barbara, Mark Benson, who had lost his partner to AIDS, said he had asked a priest where Phil was, and the priest had answered him with "a hackneyed Christian line about where the dead go. I think he quoted some line from scripture. It meant nothing to me. I realized later that I needed the priest to enter into poetry because that is where Phil is. He could have said, 'Well, Phil is at the zoo now.' Something that would clearly express the fact that Phil is gone, no longer literal, not here, not visible, but not absent, not without influence, not dead."

In New York, at an Episcopal church on Fifth Avenue, a woman said that when a friend's son committed suicide, she told the sky.

At a yoga studio, also in New York, a teacher said, "It's a struggle to find God. Some people have a kind of heart for it, but for most of us, it's a struggle. It's a struggle for me."

Sometimes people told stories that were a little too *Bible Stories Illustrated* to be quite believable, or too New Age — sunshine and ocean waves. But if you gave people enough time, the cant wore off, and the individual experience came through, often with its own ragged edges.

Once I had been to the museum in New York, I recognized what they were. Pieces of *derroteros.* Fragments of coastlines.

At the same time, texts found buried in Egypt in 1945 were finally fully translated. They dated, scholars thought, back to the second century. They are called the Gnostic gospels. Someone named Thomas wrote one that is completely different from the tone of Matthew and Mark and Luke and John. Thomas is a Zen teacher: very pure, without story. Someone named Mary wrote another, and another was written by an author named Mary Magdalene. These new gospels were discussed in some of the churches I visited, but their relationship to the four Synoptic or "certified" gospels (Matthew, Mark, Luke, John) was not discussed. And to imagine that one of them might be read on a Sunday in place of one of the four — that was really not discussed. They lived in another world, that of academic research.

Priests and ministers partially appreciated the stories told in small groups and partially condescended to them. Or what felt like condescension may have been more like confusion. The church, including me, didn't seem to know exactly what to do with them. They were the church you can't see. But they stayed with me. What I did not understand was how important they were.

One day I woke up and saw the connection between the Gnostic gospels and the stories I was hearing on the road. The Gnostic gospels were old. The stories I was hearing were new. But they had something big in common: they were witness accounts. "I saw," they said. "I encountered." "I understood." And while the Gnostic gospels were old, they were new to the church. For two thousand years, the church had relied on an approved pool of stories, the four Synoptic gospels — reliable and valuable but limited. Inside the walls of churches they were read out loud Sunday after Sunday. These new stories — the Gnostic gospels and the stories people told of their own encounters — were free range. Now what?

There was much to be said for what I saw and what I heard when I traveled, but I was missing something I did not know I was missing until it came back to me. Part of it was a particular kind of pleasure. I didn't taste my (always organic) carrots or leeks, as I ate them quickly while I made lists of the things that had not happened yet. I didn't see the tree, a beautiful Norfolk pine, in my backyard as I ducked to cross under its bough on my way to my office to write a talk or a homily or a chapter. I was not here when I was here. I was always in the world of the things not happened yet, binoculars fixed on the horizon.

Part of what I missed was something that remained nameless. I was numb in an area that was without a name. I was numb, and later, I would be raw.

I couldn't imagine stopping: when a friend said she was taking a Sabbath on Saturdays, unplugging her phone and Internet and not working and not shopping, my mind went completely blank and I asked her what she *did*. "Sometimes," she said, "I make jewelry. Sometimes I dig for potatoes. And sometimes" — here she paused — "I nap."

And like the rest of you, I lived in the United States of America in the year 2009, and I was overloaded. I have a husband who cooks and shops and cleans, unlike so many women, but I was still full of lists of things that needed to be done: the refrigerator was failing, the water heater was too old, termites had found their way into the floor near the dining room door. Our cell phones needed upgrading, our laptops were ready to explode, our garden was overgrown. The godchildren called: a girlfriend sounded unstable, a job hunt wasn't working, a marriage was proposed. Everything and everyone needed time.

I was sitting on a train talking on my cell phone to a close friend when my husband texted me, asking if I wanted to meet him at work or ride the train all the way home, and I felt as if my brain were going to divide into two halves and fall apart, like an over-ripe melon. I texted him quickly, "Will ride train," and then apologized for my abruptness, and he texted, "Sorry. U have 2b on top of everything."

I had 2b on top of everything.

Even when I didn't need to rush, I rushed. I fast-brushed my teeth, I washed the dishes so fast I dropped them, I threw laundry in the direction of the washing machine, my mind working on the things not happened yet.

A friend asked, "Why are we all in such a hurry?"

Books with advice about slowing down or living in the moment or meditation or prayer were at first attractive, then just another job. I put them down in the book-store.

I stopped listening to my neck and shoulders that spelled out IN PAIN. I registered that I was tired and pushed on. When Vincent's father died in August, my grief slowed me down but, I confess, not for long.

In September I turned sixty. There was more of my life behind me than in front. How was I to "spend" my life? But I did not ponder these things: I thought of Carissa at the window in New York and said to myself, *Let's do this forever.*

In Santa Barbara that November, planning to leave for New York, then to attend my father-in-law's memorial at a historic mining town outside Reno where he had loved to amble and record history, and then to spend Thanksgiving in San Francisco with Vincent's family, I lit the paper and kindling, sat back on my heels, and noticed the blur at the edge of my right eye. At the periphery. Very soon afterward I drowned.

CHAPTER 3

I ignored the blur. A few days later, feeling better, I got on the plane to New York, spent ten days in the apartment with Vincent, learned how to take baths in the kitchen, came back to California, boarded a plane for Reno, spread Vincent's father's ashes in the cemetery of Gold Hill, came home, and then drove to the Bay Area for Thanksgiving.

When I got back, I figured I had time, so I made an appointment with Dr. Lowe for December 1.

Our house is only a few blocks from the only hospital in Santa Barbara and its surrounding medical offices, but I drove because I planned to go down to Patagonia to work in the afternoon, and then to a book reading at my church that I was giving that night.

I felt pretty good — a little tired, I told myself, but when I got this out of the way,

I'd be fine. I measured out my life, in those days, in "getting things out of the way," and in the days between travel, and I had a good chunk coming my way. I checked in. I asked Susan, the nurse/receptionist, about her two cats. I knew about Susan's cats because I saw Dr. Lowe every three months for a checkup of an inflammatory disorder, uveitis, an inflammation of the uvea, the jelly part of the eye. I have had this disease or disorder for over twenty years in the right eye, with inflammatory episodes occurring sometimes three times a year. An underlying cause had never been found. I have a scar on my right macula from an early inflammation that causes letters to curve and crush together at the end of the eye chart. Thus I can't really read or write with my right eye. Thus I have, not to put too fine a point on it, only one "good" eye. In September 2009 I had seen Dr. Lowe, and we had both been pleased to see no evidence of inflammation.

I read the eye chart. No change from the last time I'd been there: 20/20 in the left and 20/25 minus 2 in the right.

They dilated my eyes. Susan checked the pressures. They were normal.

In about fifteen minutes Dr. Lowe, a lean Chinese American man whose uncle is a surgeon in Beijing, greeted me, swung into his chair, and asked me to put my chin on the lip of the slit lamp and look at his right ear. Then he put his eye to the lens.

The first indication that something was wrong was the length of time it took him to speak. He's a thorough man, I told myself, and waited. Then Dr. Lowe, his eye still fixed at the lens, said,

"Darn."

I half-heard him. Half of me registered that he had never said that particular word before to me, not even when there were cells in the vitreous indicating inflammation. The other half of me was rushing around like an anxious nurse, smoothing the bedcovers, restraining the patient, trying to make everything normal. *So he's never said that before,* this half of me said. *It just means you've got some inflammation. Eyedrops, and it'll all be gone by Christmas.*

He switched to the left eye and made a careful examination while my shoulders tightened. He sat back. He pushed the instrument aside. He said carefully: "You have an inflamed optic nerve."

What I knew then about optic nerves you could have put in a stamp box, but the tone was the kind you don't want to hear from a doctor. And the words *optic, nerve,* and

40

inflamed were enough to get anyone's attention. The events that followed are all shoved together in my memory, some of them collapsed and bunched and some stretched out, the first indication that I had entered another geography where the ordinary rules (gravity, time) did not apply. I can't retrieve a normal sense of the day. I must have asked him what he meant, and he said, "Just a second. We need to take some pictures."

He left the room for a few minutes, and I sat in the large examining chair while my mind attempted to grasp the words. But my mind, as it turned out, was not capable of actually "grasping" what had happened. My first feeling that things had changed was that the examining chair felt too big. It had always been too large for me — I'm five foot four and a half and had dropped to 116 pounds. (I thought I was suddenly effortlessly able to eat anything and not gain weight; I did not understand that the weight drop was part of an illness.) I felt as I had as a child sitting in a dining room chair at my aunt's farm in Wisconsin, where my feet could not touch the floor and I had to hop down to leave the room.

I wanted to jump out of the chair and run out of the room. I wanted, as I thought about it many months later, to get away from my optic nerve.

The weird feeling of wanting to remove oneself from the self, or from the thing that was wrong with the self, would crop up, in different disguises, over the next year. But when things got really scary, I didn't want to view what was wrong as a thing to be battled, overcome. The ads for Sloan-Kettering, "Dear Cancer, Good try," did not appeal to me. I understood even at the beginning that the metaphor of battle wasn't right for me.

Dr. Lowe returned and asked me if I had a stiff neck and shoulders, and when I said yes (thinking, *Who doesn't?*), he looked triumphant and said, "Maybe we've found the cause of the uveitis after all these years." He rushed out of the room again, then returned with a copy of a paper on "polymyalgia rheumatica with temporal arteritis."

"Here," he said, "you can read this later. But first" — and he called to the nurse — "let's get a visual field test and some pictures." Then he asked me, "Who is the rheumatoid doctor you are seeing?"

I told him Dr. Burks. (A young, slender woman. When we were finished with my exam, we'd talked about clothes.) Dr. Burks and I had decided a few years ago, I told Dr. Lowe, that I didn't have to see her every year for tests. Nothing had showed up. Maybe every other year, we had said. Dr. Lowe said he was going to call her. "You need some" — this phrase jolted me — *"intravenous steroids."*

I walked down the hallway and into another room, where I sat in front of a large box and put my chin on (another) platform. Susan handed me a clicker. She placed a black eye patch with an elastic band on the left eye, the good eye. I was to stare into the box, my focus fixed on a light at the center, while lights went off randomly at the periphery. I was to keep my eye on the light at the center and depress the clicker when I saw a spark of light at the edge.

I saw the dark patches on the sheet as it fed out of the machine. Very dark blotches on the lower right of the right eye. A blotch at the upper right. A stain near but not in the center. Dark areas near my nose. These were the areas where the lights had gone off and I had not seen them, the first test to verify damage in the peripheral vision. I turned away from it. Dr. Lowe walked into the room and read the results. He said (practiced, gentle): "Do you understand that this damage is permanent?"

"No," I said.

I walked down the hallway to the photo

room, and certain details caught my attention — the mind wishes to place itself anywhere but where the disaster lies. The carpet was wearing thin. A woman sat in an adjoining room calling someone, her daughter? To meet her for lunch. What was the name of the place near the hospital? she asked.

Then I was very suddenly in the little room with the fluorescein machine. They would shoot dye into my vein and then photograph my eye just as the dye entered it. I held my arm out for the IV needle, and Susan put it in, placing the tube of dye on the table beside my arm. Dr. Lowe walked in, asked if I was ready; I placed my chin on another platform and stared straight ahead at a camera. Dr. Lowe attached the tube to the IV needle and let the dye in. He shot photos of my eyes, one right after the other, the camera making a loud clacking noise. "Doing great," he said. "Just a few more."

He showed me the photos of the nerve. A stalk with a head, partly flared out. It was like a dandelion, I thought — part of it had gone to seed.

He left me there for a minute or two and then came back in the room. "I can't seem to reach Dr. Burks," he said. "Do you know where her office is?"

"Yes," I said.

"Do you mind walking over there?" he said. His tone was urgent.

I would repeat the story of the day over and over in the next weeks and months, not knowing half the time that I was repeating it, or that I had already told the person I was telling it to, and not realizing until very late the next year why I had to tell the story. To try to make sense of it. How I got here.

I put on a pair of the dark glasses they give you in eye doctors' offices that make you look like a clown and walked out the door. As I crossed the street to Dr. Burks's office, a group of doctors walked past me toward the hospital. It was, I realized, now noon. My appointment had been at nine in the morning. I had been, therefore, in Dr. Lowe's office for three hours. A couple of kids whizzed by on skateboards in front of me — just normal kids — but I drew back from them, as I had seen elderly men and women retreat from what was for them sudden danger.

Then I had an uncanny feeling of being behind a glass wall that had slid down out of the sky and separated me from the rest of the people on the street. There *they* were: walking, skating, eating, opening a window, oblivious. There I was. Carrying my eyes.

45

We were in different countries, separated by this clear, transparent wall. I could have tapped it, the way the man did in the old Colgate commercials.

The doctors and the boys on the street seemed to be moving faster than normal. They sailed past me *because they had somewhere to get to.* I knew this, because I had been them, three hours before.

My thoughts about the future, *the things not happened yet,* my ambition, my lists, my talks — *gone.* I had one goal: to get the steroids into my vein.

In the very early days of uveitis, I had had to think about, here is the word, *blindness;* I had read the statistics, looked up the studies. But as the years went by and Dr. Lowe and I *dealt with it,* I had gradually let that fear fade to where it is for most people, not on the horizon, not a possibility.

What came to my mind, as I walked toward Dr. Burks's office, were the lilacs in Abingdon Square in the Village in New York, the way they were bunched into dense deep purple clusters and then suddenly, overnight, broke out into tiny lavender blossoms. And then, unbidden, I thought of the evening I was walking near Madison Square in New York fretting over some minor offense, when I looked up and saw that the

46

winter sunset had lit up the gold spires of the MetLife Tower and the New York Life Insurance building. A trio of young men on bicycles stopped for the traffic light (probably a one-time event), and they all looked up just as I did, and one of them glanced over at me and smiled a wide grin and said, "Oh man."

As a child in New Mexico, I had been invited to piñata birthday parties. They hung the paper bird or star from the ceiling or outside, and then we kids took turns swinging at it with a baseball bat. Pretty straightforward. Only before you took a swing, they put a blindfold over your eyes.

I remembered the way the room, full of kids and adults and candles and cake, suddenly disappeared when an adult put the cloth over my eyes, and the disorientation of not only walking but swinging without being able to see. How my body disappeared. I did not allow myself to go any further with these thoughts. I had seen the dark patches on the visual field. The areas looked like puddles of dark water, and like pools, they could spread. Dr. Lowe had said, with relief, "Still on the periphery. Not in the center."

I walked up the sidewalk to a little brown-shingled cottage that Dr. Burks had made into her office and tried to open the door. It was locked. Confused, I finally read the sign on the door that said they were closed for lunch, and then I did something I have never done. I slammed on a doctor's door with my fist until a brown-haired woman wearing a white lab coat opened it. I explained the situation — my manner must have alarmed her. She went to the back of the office and returned with Dr. Burks, her blond hair cut to her shoulders, her fine-boned face a trace older. She was holding half a sandwich in her left hand with a bite taken out of it and fiddling with a small electronic thing in her right.

"My pager," she said to me, and tried to find a place to put the sandwich so she could shake my hand. "Something must be wrong with my pager."

The bite in her sandwich was the first article of what would become a collection. Next, the rumpled suit of the neuro-ophthalmologist at UCLA; the linted overcoat hanging on the hook in pulmonary at the Mayo Clinic. My eye went to the flaw in them or at least the part (bite, teeth, sandwich) that announced they were human, these . . . high priests of the country I now lived in.

48

What I didn't know until late in the game was that my little collection of human frailties in doctors was my way to counteract my automatic response to them.

"Why do I forget what I want to ask them?" I asked an acupuncturist who had been an MD but had left "Western medicine." "Why do I leave the room in a daze?"

"Witch doctors," she said. "That's the origin. You become semihypnotized in their presence. You can't help it."

This was the start of what I later identified as "the problem." Or one of "the problems." I wanted them to know everything, so they could cure me. I wanted them to be witch doctors. As time wore on, I discovered that they did not know everything, but many of them and a good part of me clung to the fantasy that they did.

Dr. Burks asked me to wait for a minute. "I'll call Dr. Lowe," she said. "I'll be right back."

I sat down in the waiting room.

When she returned, she said, "I can't do the intravenous steroids in my office today. I am sorry. I have to send you to the emergency room."

Get a blood sample first, she said, handing me a sheet for the lab.

The emergency room was just down the

block, but of course it meant that I would join the very sick, the bleeding, and the accident victims, and like many emergency rooms, it would be full of paperwork and understaffed, and getting out of it would be like getting out of jail.

As I walked through the double doors, a man wearing a bathrobe in a wheelchair was blocking the path to the reception desk. Beside the nurse at the desk was a man with his face screwed up in pain, speaking a language I had never heard, while three staff people were trying out all the languages they had among them on him. Right behind me, a man walked in with a bunch of grocery store red roses and said loudly, "If she's still breathing, that's all I care about!"

Vincent arrived as I sat there in a little plastic chair inside the emergency room door. I had waited and waited for him and had not known I was waiting for him until he walked through the double emergency room doors, and I started to cry.

He sat down and took hold of my left hand, and at the same time a nurse placed a bracelet with my name and date of birth around the other wrist.

"We have you in the system," she said.

CHAPTER 4

There are two optic nerves, one for each eye. They travel up from the spine and pass through the brain to the eyes. A neuro-ophthalmologist who examined my eyes said, "More brain tissue than nerve."

Each optic nerve has its own blood supply, from its own artery branch. Temporal arteritis is an inflammation in the arteries. (It often goes along with the disease Dr. Lowe thought I might have — polymyalgia rheumatica.) Temporal arteritis cuts off blood to the nerve, causing inflammation always, and sometimes instant blindness.

Trying to get medication to these nerves is a particular problem because of the blood/brain barrier. The brain, to preserve itself, keeps to itself. Only certain sizes of molecules are allowed through the capillaries that feed the brain, to keep bacteria, in particular, from entering the body's central system. But there are certain bacteria that "cross" the barrier — syphilis bacteria, for example, which cause the delirium that characterizes the late stages of that disease, as well as bacilli from Lyme disease.

Drugs that open up the blood vessels to the brain tend to reduce blood flow to the rest of the body.

On the Web site Uptodate, I read, "Optic neuritis is an inflammatory, demyelinating condition that causes acute, usually monocular, visual loss. It is highly associated with multiple sclerosis (MS). Optic neuritis is the presenting feature of MS in 15 to 20 percent of patients and occurs in 50 percent at some time during the course of their illness."

Vision loss can be minimal, or the disease can result in complete blindness. The average age of people who develop optic neuritis is thirty-two.

Optic inflammation can occur with and without pain. I had had none. A blur at the edge of the eye and then . . . nothing.

We went through the usual emergency room routine. A nurse led us to one of those little rooms with the shower curtain that are meant to be private; a boy lay on a cot in the hall moaning that he had "gone off the lip." I waited for the *infusion of steroids* and tried hard not to think of the blur at the periphery of my eye. They did a CT scan. The emergency room doctor said about the scan, "If there are lesions, that would be a tumor," and then asked, almost as an aside as he left the room, "Are you a drinker?" I said I liked to have a beer in the evening. My nephew called me out of the blue, and I said, "I can't talk to you right now. We are at the doctor's office," not wanting to say emergency room, and he said later, "You could have told me you were in the emergency room. It is never 'we' are at the doctor's office unless it's bad news."

The CT scan showed no lesions. The blood tests and my SED rate — the rate that red blood cells fall to the bottom of a centrifuge, and the tell-all test for most auto-immune disorders — was normal.

"Now," the doctor said, "this is beyond my expertise."

The boy in the hallway who had gone off the lip moaned and cried. I realized I had not had anything to eat since breakfast, and the nurse brought me a stale turkey sandwich. And finally the nurse hooked me up to a bag of Solu-Medrol, and it dripped into my vein. One full gram of steroids. Sixty milligrams of steroids is considered a hefty dose; one gram is a thousand milligrams.

Prednisone, as I would soon find out, is a blessing and a curse. "You will love me," Dr. Burks said the next day, "and then you will hate me." It is a most effective, quick-acting anti-inflammatory drug; and its side effects are legion: diabetes, bone destruction, cataracts, pulmonary compromise, puffed cheeks.

Vincent was preoccupied with getting the car I had left and forgotten in the parking lot at Dr. Lowe's office. I was distracted by the reading I was supposed to give that night at Trinity, my church. Both of us were concentrating on things that were very much peripheral because we could not face the reckoning in front of us. I finally called the church office, with the hand of the arm that was not hooked up to the steroid bag, explained my situation, and said something about how maybe I could make it because I hated to cancel things (this is how far gone I was), and the woman who answered the phone — I will never forget her — said, "How about postpone rather than cancel?"

They tried to keep me in the hospital overnight, to give me another infusion, but my internist, Dr. Babji Mesipam, who had somehow got wind of my presence in the emergency room, intervened and asked Dr. Burks to find out if it was possible to do

54

large infusions every twenty-four hours in her office rather than smaller ones every six hours in the hospital, and when she said she couldn't find anything against it, he sprung me. "I don't want her in the hospital overnight," Dr. Mesipam told Dr. Burks. "She'll only get sick in there."

CHAPTER 5

We came home. We live in a little yellow cottage near the hospital. We borrowed the down payment to buy our house in the late 1980s. When you imagine life in Santa Barbara, you may picture red-tiled mansions in the hills or beachfront estates, but we are writers with part-time jobs. Patagonia headquarters lies south of Santa Barbara, in Ventura, for the surf, and the real estate there is cheaper, but we thought Santa Barbara would be more cosmopolitan. We'd been living in San Francisco with a short stopover in Colorado, and when we arrived in this beautiful seaside town, we were bewildered when we could not find a place to buy an espresso. (Yes, we were from the Bay Area.) Instead, the stores sold the wares familiar to me from my childhood in other wealthy tourist towns — Aspen, Santa Fe. (My parents, in their searching, found beautiful places right before the rich found them.) The food markets in Santa Barbara were stopped in time. They sold giant bottles of gin, vodka, and whiskey placed very near the checkout stands (a kind of grab and go), and acres of Goldfish, Pepperidge Farm Milano cookies, and Scotties: salt and sweets. This town, I thought, knows how to drink and snack.

Our neighborhood must have once housed the working class, in single-wall construction cottages thrown up in the 1920s. It was charming and vulnerable to development: it had short streets lined with cork oak trees and the city's oldest park, through which ran a creek that had been lined in concrete to prevent flooding — "channelized." It lay between a hospital that was soon to triple in size and a commercial street with apartment buildings and a trailer park with a bar next to it that had long since given up on a name and simply had a pink neon sign that read lounge. Many of the people we met then called Santa Barbara paradise; I didn't know exactly what they meant. The weather? Certainly in February, when the rest of the country was suffering ice storms and frozen mud, we had freesia blooming in the rose garden next to the Old Mission. (When we flew out in January from Colorado to talk over whether we wanted to work for Patagonia, our car battery had frozen overnight, and we had to flag down a trucker to jump the car. Patagonia's owner, Yvon Chouinard, met us at the Santa Barbara airport wearing shorts.) And everywhere my eyes went, I saw beauty. But it also meant to people, I understood, that the inhabitants of paradise had to be buffed and shiny and beautiful. Once I found myself behind the glass wall, I appreciated our neighborhood's proximity to a less-than-perfect life. You could just give up and relax at the lounge.

As I walked in the door that night, our house had a forlorn, uninhabited feeling. Even in the state I was in, I could feel it. It had, without my knowing it, turned into a way station.

My diaries of that winter show an abrupt transition, or no transition at all. September through late October show lists of to-do's: Figure out how to pay taxes. Sermon: Ordinary Time. Prepare for reading. Patagonia campaigns, a meeting on wolverines, an essay on the Canadian lynx. A field report assigned to a young man who, I note now, died in an avalanche when he was skiing in the backcountry last Christmas. That diary ends with a brief notation regarding travel for a Patagonia conference: Truckee 41 degrees, 24 degrees, snow.

Then the pages are blank.

The next book starts with: "How much is the immune system 'knocked back'?" and "Vascular?" and (naïvely), "A conference call, all docs?" Lists — apricots, eggs, red peppers — healthy, "anti-inflammatory" vegetables and fruit.

Appointments written in weeks before are crossed out: *Jodie, breakfast* — crossed out. *Yoga, 10:30* — line through it. And added in: *Sansum Pharmacy, Dr. Burks, Dr. Lowe.*

I glanced at the Day-Timer lying on a chair where I had left it to go see Dr. Lowe. It was Tuesday, December 1. I still had the feeling that I should be at the reading. I should try to pull myself together.

Vincent went out to buy dinner. I lay down on our bed and felt relief to be here, in the familiar, rather than in the hospital. When you have crossed over the line that we are all safe and that everything will remain the same, normal is all you want.

Our cat, a black and gray tabby, Junior, sniffed at the bandage on my right wrist where they had put in the IV.

What fell on me was *before* and *after*. My body, which carried me around, hauled suitcases, stretched, ate, made love — its astonishing intricacies never pondered — was no longer possible to ignore. It was in the *before.* Now I was in *after,* a country that I could do nothing to leave, for which I was completely unprepared, for which I had no map. I got up and called Mark Asman, my parish priest. He told me the church had called all the people who had signed up for the reading, and he was waiting there to meet anyone who had not "heard," as he put it. Then he said he would come over. He did not make that an option.

Vincent and I ate cold salmon and asparagus, the beginning of meals from supermarkets and fast food that after a while all tasted the same but kept us going. Oz, the land of prepared food. And where the most everyday thing — the preparing of a meal — becomes too hard to accomplish.

We talked in a kind of businesslike code. He asked me what I had to do tomorrow, and I told him I had to go to Dr. Burks's office to have a second "infusion." I could walk, I said — it was only a few blocks away. He said he would still take Freya (our old Volvo) down to Patagonia.

"You might need the Prius," he said.

I did not tell him that I knew I should not drive.

In my mind was the fear of losing the remaining sight I had in my right eye, certainly. But the other fear was that this *thing* had fallen on me out of the blue, and I, and they, the doctors, did not know what it was. How had it happened? What was it? Would it strike again, in the other eye?

And then there was a third fear. Vincent's mother, Rachel, had been diagnosed with MS at nineteen. She had been sick off and on throughout his childhood. He had had to look after her, as the eldest child, or was sent to live with relatives when she was hospitalized. I could not allow myself to think about whether he might leave me, but I feared the loss of his tenderness, his attraction, our deep, mutual world. I would be a burden. As we sat at the table, I felt about a foot of distance between us, as if he had placed a ruler on the table. And the glass wall. He was not on my side of it.

I heard Mark's car on the street and went out onto the porch to wait for him. He unfolded himself from his car and brushed his hand along his shoulders. He was wearing his collar and black priest clothes. Our neighbor opened her gate as he walked by and practically curtsied. She looked up the street at me and waved, a concerned look on her face, then turned away.

I tried to light a fire, again, in a desire to be a host to a guest, not knowing, yet, not wanting to know that I was not a host, I was a patient. The fire would not light.

Mark sat down on the couch. I sat down next to him. I had known him for fourteen years; we had been through his coming out to the parish as a gay man, the ups and downs of a soup kitchen housed in the church parish hall, the deaths of my brother and parents. He was not a paragon — he was a person. He lost his temper when the tablecloths for a dinner/liturgy for Maundy Thursday were not perfectly ironed; his office was a mess; he drove volunteers too hard. But there was something about him that I knew I could count on, that was what a *priest* should be. The pain of being closeted in his youth could have led to anger, resentment, desire for retaliation. But in Mark, it made him listen. He had an ear for submerged pain. He took care of his flock; he went looking if any one of us was lost.

I told him the story. He asked me what I usually did when this kind of thing happened. I said this kind of thing had not happened to me. He asked me how I prayed when — he was careful here — something like this happened. I examined what was in my prayer repertoire. I said I went straight back to childhood, some version of "Help me." What a friend called the 911 prayer. I added that even eight hours into this, I had figured out that this version of prayer was not going to get me through this new country. I didn't tell him about the glass wall. I realized I didn't really know what prayer was. I had no practice; I had not been taught any.

A remnant of the Episcopal Great Litany went through my head: *From sin and death. Good Lord, deliver us.*

And then: *A sheep of your own flock, a lamb of your own. . . .*

And a piece of the wedding vows written by Thomas Cranmer, Archbishop of Canterbury, in the sixteenth century, that Vincent and I had spoken on a hot day in September: *With my body, I thee worship. In sickness and in health, for better or for worse.*

Parts of the large map of prayer had stuck in me, and I was glad they did, for the beauty of the prayers and what they were trying to say. For the writers who had written them. But I had no *derrotero* for Oz, nothing I could claim as my own.

Finally Mark said, "What I try to do in this kind of situation, not that this kind of thing has happened to me either, is ask myself what is real now."

I used to climb rocks, small cliffs in the mountains to the east of Santa Barbara and south in the desert at Joshua Tree. The women I climbed with called themselves the Honettes, because we were "honed women." The Honettes' idea of a biathlon was climbing and then shopping. I was once stuck in Joshua Tree in what is called an off-width crack, a crack too small to fit yourself completely into and too large to use as a handhold. I hated off-width cracks. One was invariably off balance in them, the last thing you want when you are halfway up a cliff. My right thigh was stuffed into this crack to keep me on the face while I tried to find a hold over my head and encountered only bat guano, which slowly fell into my hair.

"I can't do this!" I yelled up to my belay.

"Shut up and climb," she said helpfully.

Having no recourse, I gripped the edge of the crack with my right hand and, hoping my thigh would hold inside it, tapped my left foot along the face as if it were a blind man's cane. It encountered a small bump. I realized that if I could stick to that bump long enough, I could shift my thigh up the crack a few inches and be a little farther along, but I would have to put the weight of my left leg on the bump, and then my full weight. I would have to, in climbers' parlance, *commit.*

I looked around my living room. I was in the medical version of an off-width crack.

And what was real was that I was sitting in my living room rather than in the hospital. Vincent was in the next room, reading. Mark was sitting next to me on the couch holding my hand. I could still see.

CHAPTER 6

Mark left, and I went to bed. Junior, the cat, curled himself at my knees. Vincent snored lightly. Two bodies beside me. I tried to find words that might be a prayer. In my head were the jumbled pile of words from medicine that day that the part of me trained as a journalist was trying to get completely, accurately straight in a nonsensical exercise: *Polymyalgia rheumatoid? No, rheumatica. Optical neuritis. Solu-Medrol, which causes some patients to experience — bliss? No, euphoria. How much is one gram?*

Late in his life, my father, a lawyer and a judge, confessed to me that he didn't understand exactly what I did all day. Despite his experience writing briefs and speeches for the New Mexico Bar Association, he was not sure, he said, what a person did who had only writing to do.

We were sitting in my parents' house in Las Cruces, New Mexico, in front of a glass door that looked out on a bare lawn, the gray branches of a Russian olive tree, and a long blue sky. My mother was in Santa Barbara temporarily, living in a hotel apartment three blocks from our house. She had found a lump on her jaw, and when it didn't go away, I suggested she come out to UCLA. There a surgeon diagnosed lymphoma in about ten minutes. We brought her up to the Cancer Center in Santa Barbara, where she was undergoing chemotherapy. She was living near me; he was living in Las Cruces. He was lonely, so I went out a week before Christmas to be with him.

When I walked in the door, I breathed in the smell of Donegal tobacco. I got myself a cup of tea. My father's wispy white hair brushed his shirt collar, giving him a bohemian air. He was dressed in a tweed coat and a clean shirt and old corduroy trousers, his country gentleman's weekend clothes.

He once settled a legal case on the porch of a store in Hillsboro, a mountain village near Las Cruces, with his pants rolled up, his shoes and socks off, his feet cooling in a stream.

I'll never know whether he had it planned out — he was a careful man and a lawyer — or whether the story of his life just came up out of him, in the way a fairy tale figure who I remember swallowed the whole world and then it gushed out again, fish swimming with bugged eyes, whole towns, trains full of people, a circus tent.

He talked about the man who had brought him to AA in Union Grove in 1955. The guy had told him stories while holding his hand through the shakes.

"There was a man in a hole," the guy had told my dad. "A priest walked by and said, 'I will pray for you.' A doctor walked by and said, 'I'll try to find someone to help you.' A third man came by and jumped down into the hole with him.

" 'What are you doing?' asked the man in the hole.

" 'I've been here,' said the man, 'and I know the way out.' "

He talked about how he met my mother in 1936, when he was a student at Oxford, and she was on a tour of Europe with her mother. Among her papers after she died was a little red traveler's diary of that trip. "Met David Gallagher," she noted. "He was wearing 'Oxford bags' and a striped scarf." She was engaged to marry a young doctor who used to walk on his hands down the hallway of her father's house in Winnetka. When she got home, she broke the engagement.

They married in 1940. His best man was his best friend, who later died on a prison ship bombed accidentally by U.S. planes off the coast of Japan. They honeymooned in Jamaica, and then he joined his army unit in Tennessee. To be near him, she drove from camp to camp in a convertible they named Daisy, with Carla, the Saint Bernard, in the backseat. It was glamour all around.

The army tossed him out of the infantry because of his flat feet, and he ended up in the Judge Advocates Corps in San Antonio, Texas, and then in Dallas, where my brother, Kit, was born. After the war, they moved briefly back to Hubbard Woods, near Winnetka, and then to New Mexico.

Every now and then, while my dad and I talked, my nephew Sean would walk in from the guesthouse, and my father would lower his voice. Sean would say hi, then make himself some coffee. My dad put Sean's meds out on the counter every night and hoped he actually took them.

Sean had been the one to carry the torch of brilliance after my brother, Kit, refused to pick it up and I tried to but was, after all, a girl. Sean carried it well. He had one of the fastest minds I've ever encountered. He helped me understand IQ. His was high.

And he was sweet and incredibly funny and independent, and his mind worked with tremendous speed and clarity until it hit a train wreck called methamphetamines, LSD, a love affair gone wrong, and late adolescence. One of his psychiatric nurses once explained to me that just before you're twenty, the brain is still developing, the cells sorting themselves out. Certain "filters" are in place in childhood, she said. That was the best way to describe it. And gradually those filters are lifted, one by one, as you grow into early adolescence and then late adolescence and then your twenties. If all goes well, the filters are all up and everything's fine, and you've got a working adult brain. And if it doesn't? You get a boy who at nineteen started talking to me on the phone from Santa Cruz, where he was a student in psychology at the university, about how the cat at the bar he was working in was telling him about its life.

I rescued a little pocket calendar from his possessions after he spent an ill-fated sojourn in Santa Barbara. Notations in it stopped, precisely, in August 1985, a few months after that first disturbing phone conversation and at the point he completely lost his mind. Or rather, most of it. His memory is locked in that year, or before it, but not after. The friends then are still fresh in his mind, the books he was reading (Fromm, Erickson, Hume) as if on his current shelf, the car he wanted and the one he drove. And everything after that, which is now everything over twenty-seven years, is scrambled, hazy, delusional, things having taken place in the half-light of another planet that he knows is not as real as the one he left that year, but one he can't quite leave, can't quite find the right rocket to send him back.

I tried to visit him in his studio every day I was there that December. The single room was dark with tobacco varnish and cigarette ash. Stacks of books like Kant and Nietzsche and James were covered in dust, books he once read with pleasure and understanding. *Squalid* doesn't actually cover it, more like *unable to concentrate long enough to see what was around him.* My father and I always lowered our voices when Sean came in to make coffee, spreading coffee grounds in the kitchen, talking to "Jenny."

My dad and I knew, I think, that this was our last chance. He died the next year, just after September 11, 2001.

When he asked me about writing, I very much appreciated that he had asked me, and was moved that he had waited this long

71

to ask. I told him I got up in the morning, had breakfast, and read the paper, then went to my studio in my sweats and rewrote what I written the previous day.

I told him that Judith Thurman, contracted to write a biography of Colette, was so intimidated by her subject that she refused even to turn on her computer for a year, and that I too was sometimes unable to put words on paper, or was unable to stop myself from putting too many words on paper and then did not know how to get rid of them. Or I stared paralyzed at the page as the beautiful thing I had in mind turned into a monster. But writing, I said, was the way I made sense of my life and discovered what I was thinking. I compulsively make notes. I spend days and sometimes months mulling the strings of events, facts, thoughts, random encounters, and journal entries to discover what binds them together. What story is hidden in them. Writing is certainly a voyage of discovery. It is sometimes a shipwreck.

I tried to find the right word, I told him, for the thing it signified. The right word is like a piece of a jigsaw puzzle that perfectly slips into place. The right word leads to the next right word and makes things and ideas spring to life. The wrong word — how I

would learn this when I fell into Oz —
deadens and destroys. In the beginning,
John's gospel says, was the word.

I finally said that George Orwell compared
writing a book to a long bout with a painful
illness, hoping to make him laugh. But he
didn't, and I realized that he was thinking
of my mother.

The next day was Christmas Eve, and I
asked Sean if I could go with him to mid-
night Mass at his (Roman Catholic) church.
As we approached the adobe cathedral, men
were lighting votive candles in little brown
sacks weighted with sand along the side-
walks and at the arched entrance. *Lumi-
narios,* lit on Christmas Eve to make a path
for the Christ child to find his way home.

We entered a dense mass of women and
children and men. I remember nothing of
the service except for the middle, before
communion, when Sean stood up and
turned to me and said, "Peace," and we
hugged each other. Then one by one, people
came up to us and said, "Sean, peace be
with you," and he wished them, by name,
peace back, and introduced each person to
me. I stood there in the sea of my nephew's
church all around him, despite his hair, his
elephants, and his voices.

My father was waiting up for us. We stood

in the kitchen. Sean went out to his studio, got his guitar, and came back. He plucked out the tune while my father and I sang "Silent Night."

Just after I visited my dad, I ended the arduous business of discerning a "call" to the Episcopal priesthood. I had been inspected, examined, dissected. I had met with a group of four people at Trinity for a year in a little upstairs room at the church with lumpy sofas and old leaded windows that cranked open. We sat in silence, "discerning" or listening, for the voice of something other. Mark Benson, one of the committee's members (the man who hoped his partner had gone to the zoo), said that one of the sessions felt like the movie *Poltergeist,* "with things flying around the room in slow motion."

I met with another group in another church where I volunteered for a year. I talked with diocesan boards in Los Angeles and addressed my lack of proper credentials with seminaries and, most memorably, took the Minnesota Multiphasic Personality Inventory — a series of statements with which you agree or disagree.

"Most of the time I wish I were dead."

"I am afraid of using a knife or anything

very sharp or pointed."

"I hear strange things when I am alone."

When I was finished, I felt as if I had been run through a car wash, and while the church was clear that I was indeed called to be a priest, I was not. I hesitated. I, who don't usually procrastinate, procrastinated. Finally, after all that work and time (not only mine but so many others'), I said no. I hoped I wasn't saying no to God (famously a bad idea). I knew I was saying no to the priesthood of the institutional church. The priesthood of the visible collar. The professional priesthood. I was clear about that no.

And a few other people were clear about the no as well. I led a retreat at a local monastery, about a year after I decided not to go to seminary, with the people from the church where I had worked during my ministry study year. Saturday evening, one of the men who had been on my "discernment committee" at that church walked up to me, after we'd both had a beer, and said, "You sure look a lot happier than you did when you were working with us."

"Was it that obvious?" I asked him.

"Yes," he replied.

I was never quite sure entirely, in the end, why I stopped. The lingering question was: If I am saying no to that priesthood, to what am I saying yes? There was something on the periphery that I couldn't make out. A door closes and another one opens, said a friend, but it's hell in the hallway.

Vincent doesn't go to church, but during the time I was "discerning," he said he was not so worried about a difference in belief between us as he was about the demands of the professional priesthood: he did not see himself as a minister's wife. And he was not so sure it was the right choice for me: when I worked in the soup kitchen at the church, he pointed out, I came home light and cheerful. When I came home from a church meeting during the year I was discerning the vocation to priesthood, he said, "You are full of planning and intrigue."

"I know you can't do it without me," he said one day, "and I don't wish it for me. But it's also not what I wish for you."

As I traveled down the road toward the vestments and the collar, the evening meetings and the Sundays taken over by church events, the gulf between us widened. But one night I led a service of Taizé, from a community in France that has formed itself around simple songs sung in Latin and a lot of silence. The leaders there devised these liturgies to reach the thousands of young people who come to Taizé speaking different languages.

The church was dark. Vincent decided only at the last minute to join us. Afterward he said he liked it. It was to him, a combination of "Quaker and Catholic."

"It's funny," he said. "I can't sing 'Lord, I adore you,' but I can sing *Adoramus te domine*." That night I began to see, dimly at first, then more clearly that part of the reason I had decided not to be a priest was because of words. Partly because of being a writer of words.

I preached on and off during the years of discernment, and one Sunday in Santa Barbara, one of my closest friends, Jodie Ireland, came to hear me. Her mother had just died. She told me later she began to cry at some point during the service. Churches are one of the few places left where you can publicly and honorably cry.

"Then you stood up," she said, "and started saying, 'I believe in God the Father, and his only Son,' and I didn't believe it, so I stayed put." (She didn't come back.)

She was referring to the Nicene Creed, which begins: "I believe in God, the Father Almighty, maker of Heaven and Earth. I believe in Jesus Christ, his only Son. I believe that he came down from Heaven . . ." I had been standing up and saying the creed since I joined St. John's Cathedral. I can recite it like the poems I memorized in the fourth grade. But I took note that Sunday that one of my dearest friends found the words of the creed the thing that divided her from the other people in the church, and from me, when she had, moments before, found a place to grieve.

Shortly thereafter I was at breakfast one morning at an Episcopal monastery in the hills above Santa Barbara, and I asked a table full of priests what they thought about the creed. Three of them said they only *mouthed* parts of it. One of them, a young man from Los Angeles, said he was entirely frustrated with it because on Sunday morning he didn't have time to explain to the new people who might be there out of deep need or longing or because they had experienced something they didn't understand, that the "Virgin Mary" in the Nicene Creed was a metaphor. I thought of Jodie.

"The church is better at telling people what the church believes than at eliciting from people what they believe," said Gary Hall, dean of the Washington Cathedral in Washington, D.C. "I think that anyone who gets themselves and their family up and goes to church in the face of so many attractive alternatives must have access to some deep truth or experience of God that they are seeking to make sense of in community. The church responds by boring them out of their minds and telling them what we think is shameful."

The words of the creed were written down in Nicaea, in what is now Turkey, in the fourth century, at a meeting organized by the Roman emperor Constantine, a new and opportunistic convert to Christianity. Constantine wanted to bring some order to the many stripes and communities that made up this now-popular religion. And because of that, a lot of things changed:

"In the changed world of the fourth century, . . . when Christians ceased to be liable to occasional persecution and became instead *the favoured cult of the Roman empire,* the character of their Eucharistic worship also changed," says Paul Bradshaw, an authority on the Eucharist (communion). "Celebrated now in large public buildings, it took on the style of imperial court ceremonies and incorporated features drawn from the pagan religions around, of which it saw itself as the true fulfilment."

Before this meeting at Nicaea, there had been no creed, no special buildings for worship. There had been instead gatherings of people in houses, around a table.

The meeting at Nicaea and the creed itself were the beginning of the large map of Christianity. It was an effort to gather up disparate strands, different stories, a ragtag band of men and women who were following what was a memory and to make them into One. Out of Nicaea came the ideas — "God, the Father Almighty," "Jesus Christ, his only Son," "He was born of the Virgin Mary," "He ascended into Heaven."

What had been a messy group of followers on a road of discovery suddenly became the empire's religion, linked, fatefully, to a state, to power, and to conquest.

It is the map that people outside the church think all of us inside the church believe. They think we believe that Jesus is God's only son. They think we believe that his mother was a virgin. As the Red Queen says to Alice, "Six impossible things before breakfast." After all, that's what we stand up and say Sunday after Sunday. Not being able to swallow these rather hard-to-take ideas, they turn away. And wonder how otherwise intelligent people could believe such things. "You're smart," said the dean of Grace Episcopal Cathedral in San Francisco, her tongue firmly in her cheek, to the performance artist Anna Deavere Smith,

"How come you're religious?"

Jesus never said a word about being God's *only* son, nor made mention of his mother's sexual history. These are the words placed in his mouth by those who wished to smooth out a fragmented story, a bumpy road, pointing, now I see, in an entirely different direction.

In my travels, I talked to sophisticated Christians in Georgia and, in Berkeley, to yearning secularists. A young couple asked Vincent and me to preside at their wedding; another asked me to baptize their baby boy, outside, by the ocean, not in a church. People were in need, I could see, and sometimes the church filled it (where else was my nephew welcome?), but many times it did not.

I kept going to church, one foot inside it, one foot outside, and on the talk circuit, trying to find the words that would reach those inside but not sound too crazy to those outside it. I tried to explain that there were a bunch of us who went to church who were not filled with passionate certainty; nor were we stupid. We knew, for example, that the gospels were written long after Jesus's death; that Paul's letters came first, before the gospels; that scholars had figured out, more or less (mostly less), at least some

81

of the words that might authentically be those of Jesus and those that were attributed to him hundreds of years after his death.

All this fascinating information — the historical Jesus, the time lag in the writing of the New Testament, the Gnostic gospels — was not exactly trumpeted from the rooftops in churches. It was, rather, whispered in the back alleys. The church, once it drew its large map, worried about what would happen to the laity's "faith" if we knew too much.

Now I lay in bed with medical terms mixed with fragments of the old words of the church's prayers, hoping they would lead me away from fear and into relief. I had no experience with what was prayer and what was not prayer. What floated into the middle of this heap of words was a strange image: frogmen, swimming in my eyes, were working very hard to link together cables, like those huge things that hold up the Golden Gate Bridge. (I have not yet discovered where this image came from.) I was entranced. They swam, seemingly without my assistance: pulled, captured a stray strand, linked it to another, bolted it in.

What is in charge of healing? I thought. How does the body know what to do?

What followed the frogmen in my mind was the line from "Suzanne": "and when he saw for certain only drowning men could see him." I've drowned, I thought, but there's something in the water with me. And then I thought, Will I see him?

CHAPTER 7

In the morning, I started what would be the routine for the next three days, adapting overnight, as human beings do, to complete change. One day I was going to work, driving, writing, producing. The next day what had been on my calendar was replaced with one appointment: Dr. Burks's office, IV. I had talked about stopping my bizzy, crazy life. Now it — I — was stopped.

I had breakfast, did not read the newspaper. Vincent went to work, looking haggard and determined. I managed to respond to a few e-mails and then went back to bed. In the early afternoon I walked three blocks to Dr. Burks's office. I noticed on the way signs that said "restoration" work would begin soon on the creek that ran through our park. I thought I might check that out, one day.

I sat in Dr. Burks's uncomfortable wicker and wood chairs and did not read *Arthritis*

Today. Fairly soon her nurse, Dianna, called me into a small room with two lounge chairs in it, hooked me up to the IV without hurting me, and covered me with a ratty red fleece blanket. I sat in the chair with the IV taped to my wrist, steroids dripping from a bag, drop by drop, down a clear tube, into my vein. I alternated between dozing and staring into space. I hadn't brought a book or a magazine with me because I was afraid to read. I didn't own an iPod.

On the second day, a woman slightly older than me joined me in the room for her infusion, in the next chair. We chatted about what our Thanksgivings had been like, and the weather. I had so far not met another inhabitant of this country, or at least a person who might live there, so I felt a kinship with her, although she looked — in her pressed shirt, bright trousers, and neat, coiffed hair — the complete opposite of me. She asked me what had gone wrong, and I told her about the nerve. She didn't say what was wrong with her. Her infusion finished before mine, and as she left, she said, "Think positively." It was, of course, well meaning: an attempt to help. I had said some version of it myself or been on the brink of saying it ("Things will get better") to someone recovering from surgery or sick with the flu in an effort — I thought then, before arriving here in this country — to give them a bromide, to offer a way out of where they were (as if they hadn't thought of ways out themselves). But when I heard her words, even before she was out the door, I felt more alone. Think positively? I could barely think at all.

On that second day, the routine was broken because the pharmacy didn't deliver the Solu-Medrol to Dr. Burks's office in time for my appointment. The pharmacy staff person ("What is your date of birth?") said they didn't get the fax ordering it until after eleven, and so they couldn't order it from their supplier. I asked to speak to the pharmacist, who said that she would try to find it from the hospital next door and call me back. When she did, asking my date of birth, she said she had ordered two bags because then I would have only one co-pay. This combination of mix-up followed by kindness was, I would soon understand, common in the medical world. I rode a roller coaster of panic and confusion, followed by gratitude. The number of times things went wrong was plenty scary; the number of times people were willing to run to fix them was extraordinary.

Vincent came home after work and a visit to the gym. My mind was full of Solu-Medrol deliveries, the fleece blanket, Dianna's skill. Vincent lived in the country of e-mail, editing, and writing and of the body's trustworthy dependability. He'd picked up a chicken cooked in orange sauce, and I exclaimed over how delicious it was (see "steroids: euphoria") until he glanced over at me, and I understood I was not acting normally. We looked at each other across the border, warily. I felt more dependent on him than I had ever felt or ever thought I would feel. He said something about Christmas, and I realized I didn't know what day it was.

After the steroid infusions, Dr. Lowe planned to measure my sight and visual field again. My eye still had the blur. Deep in my brain, there was a voice saying, *You put off seeing the doctor . . . you put off seeing the doctor . . .*

Meanwhile I now had three doctors: Dr. Mesipam, my internist, who had sprung me from the hospital; and Dr. Burks and Dr. Lowe, who were individually trying to figure out what had caused the inflammation in the nerve. Dr. Burks was worried about temporal arteritis, the inflammation of the arteries, which usually occurs in people older than me but could happen to a person my age. The way to discover temporal arteritis is to do a biopsy of the temporal artery. I did not allow myself to imagine what this meant. Temporal arteritis is an autoimmune disease, as is polymyalgia rheumatica, which often goes along with arteritis. Uveitis, the eye disorder I'd had for years, is also an autoimmune response. My mother had had an autoimmune disease, and my doctors had been interested when I noted that on my medical history, but a connection between her disease and mine had not been established.

In the days ahead, in visits to various medical offices, I came across other people besides the other infusion patient. In my previous life, I had behaved as if I were so temporarily in this medical zone that the other people in the waiting room were not quite real. I passed a magazine; I commented on the weather. I was so sure I would never be *really sick* that I saw no need to recognize the human person sitting near me, *Ladies' Home Journal* and the big-type *Reader's Digest* between us. Now I studied them. When I went back to Dr. Lowe's office, my second visit back after the initial disaster, an elderly couple were sitting across from me. She was clearly the patient, a little dazed, tired, her eyes sometimes drifting, lids closing, her sweater and skirt thrown together. Her husband, on the other hand, personified the word *dapper,* in a three-piece suit and polished shoes reading *Money* magazine. He was managing to sit in such a way as to be separate from her, even leaning away from her body. His clothes, his concentrated reading, his manner all said, *I am not one of you.*

I watched her fall gracefully to sleep. I identified with her, this worn, vulnerable woman who was sick.

Susan led me to the small room, where I once again propped my chin on the plastic cup and peered into the white box. She put a black patch over my left eye and the clicker in my right hand and told me to stare straight ahead with my right eye at the orange light. (Later Susan gave me one of the eye patches they used for the visual field test, and I wore it when typing to give the right eye a rest. I caught myself in the mirror with my eye patch rakishly in place; I was a writer pirate.)

I was so tired I felt nauseous. The lights

went off in a fog. When the paper rolled out from the machine, there were more dark patches in the bottom quadrant, creeping toward the center.

Dr. Lowe said it was not a surprise. "Sometimes it takes this long for the assault on the nerve to show itself."

It's worse, I thought. They told me it would not get worse once the steroids kicked in. Dr. Burks had said, "That would be extremely rare."

I asked Dr. Lowe if this damage was also permanent. And how had it gotten worse?

He said carefully, "It takes a while, sometimes, for the damage to show up."

I called Vincent on my cell phone as I walked home. I was crying. He said, in a voice that was new to me, that was meant to anchor me and did, "You'll have to live with ambiguity. You'll have to live with that for a while."

Dr. Lowe and Dr. Burks agreed that I should take 60 milligrams of prednisone (the pill version of a steroid) a day and then, very gradually, begin a taper. He would measure the visual field once a week.

The next week I had the scheduled biopsy of the temporal artery. I managed not to imagine what it would be like, and despite the fact that no anesthesiologist called me, I consoled myself that they would put me under.

Vincent and I walked over to the clinic and met Mark Asman in the waiting room. (The term *waiting room* I collected as part of my new vocabulary. The name we use without thinking that connotes exactly what it is.) Mark is practiced at passing the time in medical zones, and he led us in making up waiting room magazine titles:

WAITING ROOM
LACK OF IRONY TODAY
REAL ESTATE GALORE

He asked me if I wanted him to come into the treatment room when the nurse called, and I said yes. I wanted him around as long as he was willing. Vincent remained in the waiting room.

The nurse said of course he could come in and she would tell him when he had to leave. She led us down a short hallway to a small, sterile white room with a very narrow combination lounge chair and cot in one corner. Odd music came from speakers in the ceiling. I had a momentary memory of the brief late-1960s BBC series *The Prisoner,* when Patrick McGoohan is caught in a

91

model "village" and a voice says periodically, "Number nine."

The nurse left us for a few minutes, and Mark and I stood next to a cabinet filled with sterile bandages and syringes trying to find a place to put our eyes. The nurse returned with a small bundle of things, all of which looked scary: sharp silver scalpels, bandages, and something that looked like dental floss and must have been sutures.

It will only be a few minutes, she said. The doctor is cleaning up. I had an image of a man with blood up to his elbows washing it off in a trough.

Mark said, "I'd like to pray." The nurse was standing at the threshold about to pass through the door when she stopped, turned, and said with hesitation, "May I join you?"

"Of course," we said. And Mark added, "The more the merrier. May I ask you your name?" She said it was Marci.

The three of us held hands. Mark let a long moment of quiet pass. And then he said, "We ask you, Creator, to be with us today and especially with Nora and with the surgeon and with Marci to relieve us all of anxiety." This was a prayer, I thought. It said exactly what I needed to hear.

Mark said, "Amen," and Marci said. "That was really nice." And later when

Mark left, she said to me, with admiration in her voice: "What denomination is he?" I wondered what she would have thought had she known that Mark was gay. And that that part of his character — his warmth, his capacity to include a stranger — came from what he had made of vulnerability.

Later she would say she prayed every morning with her children, and I would wonder if she was a fundamentalist — Christians are deeply divided because of the horrors of combining politics with religion — but then it did not matter. It did not matter a whit. What mattered was that someone from the medical world was willing to join us in a human activity other than cutting into flesh and carrying bandages, that the "practiced manner" of the medical world, often distant, detached, was dropped. And later still I thought, if she prayed every morning with her children, maybe she knew something about prayer.

Mark left, and Dr. Cizek walked in. His manner was brisk. He told me to lie on my left side, that I would feel a prick as he injected something to deaden "the area." He did this with dispatch. I was in a little nightie with a blanket over me, and I felt, as in the chair at Dr. Lowe's office, like a child. Marci sat next to me. Dr. Cizek and I chatted about his name, Czech, and my last visit to Prague, as the deadening made its way into the "area," namely my temple. Then he said, less briskly, more seriously, "Now we're going to have to be quiet, and you will have to lie very still," and I realized he was going to cut into my artery, and if I moved . . .

The urge to move was always there right under the grip of not moving.

I smelled burning, and he said, "That is what you think it is."

I lay completely still for twenty-five minutes while he took sections of my artery, cauterized the edges, did not cut through the artery and cause me to bleed to death, and then, with a word about how I would feel a tugging, stitched me up. Marci held still. She kept me still.

Then, with a few words about when I could take off the bandage and when the stitches would "fall off," I was spilled out into the waiting room where Vincent took my hand. His expression told me I did not look good. He took me home.

The transition from the biopsy room to my house felt as strange as if I had been in an instant transporter. I was in one world: a sterile room, a white gown, a doctor who cauterized flesh, the fear of a slipped knife, and then I was back in my dining room with my grandmother's Biedermeier dining table and chairs and a teapot, still warm, that I'd made to cheer myself up even though I could not drink it until after the biopsy was over. My desire to be "normal," I understood, was so powerful that it rendered the experience in the clinic to a place in my mind where it had not actually happened.

I wanted a connection between the two besides the one embodied in me. I thanked Marci again for stepping out of her role as "nurse" and into "human," by joining us to pray. She was the other connection, besides me, between two increasingly separate worlds.

In the next week, in the middle of the nights, I reviewed the days. I know insomnia, but this was not it. My thoughts needed the night, its quiet, the unconscious person next to me, the lack of distraction. In those early days, I woke up, partly because of the steroids and partly because I had to go over, absorb, not make sense of, not yet, but bring closer, the days. Because the days were spent in the unfamiliar country, behind the glass wall. I had to acquaint myself and interpret the huge presence of medicine, medical systems, clinics, doctors — a place

I thought I had known but did not. I had to start to draw a map. I had to learn its words. Oz, as it turned out, would exact its own language.

One night, as I lay awake, the day's words pouring through me (*lower quadrant, vasculitis, kidney failure*), it started to rain. Rain in California is almost always a welcome relief; we live in a desert, with a wet season only in the winter months. In New Mexico, rain was never taken for granted. At first it was a drip drip, then a kind of clatter, and then a whoosh as the gutter near our bedroom window poured out. I lay awake, relieved of fear and dread for a few minutes because of the rain. The rain came down, falling evenly. I could count on it. I smelled the fresh air through the open bedroom window. It would water everything; nothing I could do or not do would change it.

As I listened to the rain, I understood that I was, more or less, in the present. In what was real now, as Mark would say. And I was not oblivious to my experience of the world. I was in the world, and it was raining. I felt my smallness, a small thing, in a bed, with the large rain all around me. Ever since I was a child, I've had these moments when I sense the large world just briefly, all that is, outside me. It doesn't seem to matter what

I am doing or where I am; I get this sense of how big it all is, a globe spinning through space. And with this apprehension comes the word *miracle.* Grizzlies, salmon, bees, sunflowers, sand, oceans; Marci, the nurse; Vincent, granite ledges, an unending flow.

I had been skipping over the present in my efforts to work through the list of those *things not happened yet.* I so regularly skipped over the present that I thought it had no value. What had value was the next thing. And the world? I passed *through* the world, barely glancing left or right.

But that night, in the rain, I thought that the present had something in it, and the word that came to my mind was so generic it hardly matched what I felt. The present had *information* in it.

If you stayed in the present, if you paid attention thoroughly to the now, what it had in it might come to you. And if you did not pay attention to the present, you might miss essential *information* that might be exactly what you needed. More than what you needed. Janusz Szuber wrote:

The real, hard as a diamond,
was to happen in the indefinable
Future, and everything seemed
Only a sign of what was to come. . . .

Now I know inattention is an unforgivable
   sin.
And each particle of time has an ultimate
   dimension.

Each particle of time. Has an ultimate
dimension.

About five days into what I now called *it*,
Jodie (my friend who had come to hear me
preach) called to ask me if she could do
something for me. I had talked to her on
the phone; she had the bare outlines of what
had happened — I could sense in her voice
that she was trying to figure out what. She
would bring me something, she said, or we
could go somewhere. She would drive. Her
voice was anxious. She and two other
women were my close, dear friends in town.
She was also more than a friend; she was a
comrade. We had been in a trench together.
   It was July 2008. I was packing for a vacation to a valley in northern Washington
state, thinking of wilderness hikes and my
cousins' good company. The phone rang. I
picked it up. Jodie said, "Something has
happened to Frank. I'm driving to the
hospital. Will you meet me there?"
   I put down the phone and ran. When I
got there, Jodie was sitting outside at a table

near the emergency room. As I walked toward her, a fireman, a friend of mine, ran from his car to meet us. Jodie's husband, Frank, had been surfing off a wild coast north of the city, alone. But other men on the beach had looked up at some point and realized he was facedown in the water. They paddled out. They brought him in. They called 911. One of them was a doctor, and he tried to revive Frank. A helicopter flew up, and now it was flying back. It would land at a school nearby, and Frank would be put in an ambulance. Jodie and I sat at the table holding hands. It was very quiet. When we saw the ambulance, we stood together holding on to each other at the gaping hole in the hospital wall that was the driveway. A chaplain, who had joined us, said to me when we saw Frank on the gurney, "This does not look good." I remember a feeling of ice passing through my body.

In the days that followed Frank's death, I tried and tried to find ways to ease Jodie's suffering. Every day it was like a pile of sand that I tried to climb, and every day more of it slid down and I found myself at the bottom again. One memory in particular stands out. I was with her in her bedroom on the day of Frank's memorial as she sat with her children and his ashes. They were dividing them up, some to be cast into the ocean, some to be kept in a jar. She looked up at some point, and I looked into her eyes, and in them was a terrible blank horror and sorrow and rage. I could not take it in. What did I do? I looked away.

I told Jodie I wanted to walk on the beach. This sounded almost unattainable, but I wanted to try. The beach in December in Santa Barbara is often beautiful and deep. The water recedes, exposing the sand and rock, and the air is clearer than in the summer (when fog often comes in early and hugs the coast).

Jodie picked me up, and we drove to Hendry's Beach, where locals often walk their dogs, and were soon out on the sand. I felt excited, as if I were on an exotic trip. I had not been on the beach since "it." She settled herself on my right. We talked preliminaries. I looked ahead as she talked, enjoying the company of my beloved friend, and then I suddenly realized she was a blur, a shadow, a watery shape, coming into and out of the field, sometimes suddenly, sometimes not at all. I could no longer see her on the periphery of my vision. I had not known what exactly I had lost, and now I knew. I might lose some more, too — this came at me at the same time. I almost cried out.

Then Jodie said, "What are you afraid of?"

"Going blind," I said.

"And then?" she said.

"I don't know," I said. "I don't know if I could live."

CHAPTER 8

It was now mid-December. Vincent's family by tradition comes to our house for the holidays, and we would host Vincent's stepmother, her brother, and her nephew. Because Vincent's father had died so recently, in August, the gathering was all the more weighted. These were people I loved. But how we were to manage the day-by-day while I was living in another country, we had not allowed to enter our conscious minds. I made lists and discarded them. I could not shop. Our beautiful and spirited cousin, Claire, got engaged to her Matt, a steelhead biologist, the exactly right man for her. I missed both the small family dinner and the larger celebration.

I was off the intravenous steroids and on the pills. I looked at the bottle every morning with distaste and then swallowed six round tablets, which rapidly puffed up my cheeks and made a small hump on my back.

I had never had to take a prescription medicine for more than a few days. I had never had side effects. I felt old and ugly.

Vincent was the merest distance away.

One Saturday morning, over breakfast, I said to him off-handedly that I'd read somewhere that when men got sick, their wives took care of them. And when women got sick, their husbands left.

"I'll be leaving in a few weeks," he said, not looking up.

"Thank you for the warning," I replied, same tone.

"I thought I would leave before Christmas," he said, "because then you could forget about it and go to Paris."

"I appreciate your thoughtfulness."

"No problem," he said, using the phrase common in California, a phrase we had often discussed: did it mean "thank you" or "don't mention it" or "yes, it was a problem, but I can cover it"?

We went on with the day as if no conversation had taken place, and in the afternoon Vincent proposed that we go together to buy a Christmas tree. I agreed, but before we got in the car to go to our usual lot, we sat down in the dining room.

I said something about how I was beginning to understand the value of the present.

I could catch, without his having to say anything, that this was not a conversation he wished to have, but I kept on going in an effort to reach him, across the gulf or the twelve inches that was between us — it did not matter how large or long — me on Saturn, he on the planet Earth. I would make a tether with words, I thought, but the only ones that came out of my mouth sounded, as I heard myself speak them, like those from a New Age fluff head. "The present," I said, "is all we have."

He was lying on the window seat. I was sitting at the dining room table.

I said, "It has been a drag . . . but the present is . . . full." I ground to a halt.

Vincent said, "The present isn't great for me. I'm getting nothing from this. I'm completely exhausted, and all I want is to go and get a damn tree."

I took this to mean that he really planned to leave me.

I remembered how I had felt when he got his right hip replaced. (His hip ball had never really developed, causing him pain throughout his life.) I had to leave at five a.m. to drive from a friend's house in the Hollywood Hills to the hospital in Santa Monica — he wanted me to be there as he woke up. The traffic always stalled me, and he was always hurt because I was always late. Once we were home, I helped him on with his blood-clot-prevention stockings every morning, got his breakfast, brought him the newspaper. I put everything I could think of at counter height the day I left for New Mexico for three days because at the same time my brother was dying of cancer in Socorro. I discovered how hard it is to be a nurse, and how even the smallest things (helping someone with stockings) become too much to bear because they are on a list with ten other things and your own full-time life, and how exhausted you are, how there is no "gift."

Fighting back tears and fear, I tried to say something about understanding what he must be feeling (which sounded like something out of *Marriage Counseling for Dummies*), but soon I began to rant about how I was the one who'd had to go to all the doctors' offices and have a temporal artery biopsy and would possibly lose my sight. (We would call this, later, "playing the sick card.") I stopped.

When we first moved in together, in that state of passionate love that made everything, even traffic jams and moving boxes, into bliss, we got all our possessions, finally, into the house in the Berkeley Hills with views of the Bay Bridge and the Golden Gate (well beyond our means) and, exhausted, had a huge fight. Furious, I took a look at this man, the guy I had thrown my lot in with, and realized it was all a big mistake and I should leave him right then (I was twenty-nine). But before I did, I called an old friend. She said, "Go out on the deck and stand there and say together, 'It's not what it was cracked up to be.' "

Over twenty-five years later, we looked at each other in the dining room and silently walked to the car and got in. Floating over our heads was all that was not and could not be resolved: Vincent's surprise and resentment and exhaustion and guilt; my surprise and fear and paranoia and exhaustion and guilt and isolation. The anxiety over the upcoming family visit. Christmas itself.

Vincent said, "I didn't mean to hurt you."

"I get that," I said. "I was hurt, be that as it may,"

Our particular Christmas tree lot is on a fairground run by a family that seems only once removed from the drug trade, and this year they had decided to include karaoke with the buying of a tree. When we drove up, a young black man was singing "White Christmas." The owners, husband and wife, were sitting in lawn chairs smoking and looking as if they'd rather be driving back to Oregon, while their teenage son rummaged in their trailer, soon to emerge with a chain saw.

I got out of the car feeling suddenly cheerful. We walked around, as was our habit, to different parts of the lot finding trees we liked and calling out to each other their better attributes. This one is very healthy, I said, and then pondered my choice of words. We usually emerged from the forest with our leading candidates and then negotiated. Or argued until one of us gave in. The wandering through the trees in their stands was immediately soothing to me. We might last through buying the tree. We had a *routine.*

I found a round (healthy) tree, my candidate.

Vincent found a very tall thin tree, a spruce, on sale. I did not like the tree. I thought it would look like a large toothpick in the dining room. I wasn't even sure it would fit. But I looked at him, and some part of me, so absorbed in life on my side of the wall, so consumed by my own fear and dread and illness, found a way out and said that I thought the tree might really work. He looked pleased. The teenage boy, happily wielding the saw, cut the base to fit our stand and helped load it into the car, and we drove home.

We hauled it out of the car and managed to carry it up the driveway. Vincent opened the French doors of the dining room/living room wide, and we got it in. I felt fit and hearty, a woman who could carry half a tall tree. I crossed the fingers of my heart, and we stood it up.

It was, of course, the most beautiful tree we had ever had. It suited the dining room perfectly; its height reached into the pitch of the ceiling. Vincent looked like a man who had conquered K2; I managed to congratulate him without sounding peevish. The present, I figured, did not have to be discussed or made holier than it was. It was here, in all its hereness, tree lots, karaoke, a chain saw, a tired man and a sick woman bound by vows written down in 1549 by a new archbishop who loved a woman and was alive to words, a man who understood what is lovely and simple and safe to say, as a feeling from the heart becomes a wild dare when spoken as a promise. We had said "in sickness and in health" then, and now the dare had presented itself.

CHAPTER 9

Books were to my family's house like beds and stoves, the most basic items, necessary for survival. When I sat with my father that last Christmas, behind him on the shelves were the titles I had read all my life, lined up like old friends: Emma Goldman's *Living My Life,* A. E. Housman's poems, Winston Churchill's *The War Years.*

My parents read to me nearly every night before I went to sleep. The characters in those books, whether real or imagined — Laura Ingalls Wilder in *The Little House in the Big Woods;* Ratty and Moley in *The Wind in the Willows;* Dickon and Mary in *The Secret Garden* — were alive. I knew they were different from the people who lived around me, in the flesh, but when my mother read to me the opening of *The Secret Garden,* I saw Mary, a little girl — pale, angry, alone in the middle of a big, empty house in India, with only a small green snake for company. I more than saw her, I knew her. She was me and not me. I didn't question this, didn't ask myself how it happened. I had an imagination, and my imagination met the imagined world of writers. Our minds seek, long for, must have, a story.

The imagination has no boundaries. It seeks the dark as well as the light. It loves the shadowed, the profane, the perverse, as much as the bright, the forgiving, the acceptable. During the Spanish Inquisition, the state and church (Queen Isabella and King Ferdinand and a pope under pressure from the two monarchs) censored Ovid, Rabelais, and Dante, but many scholars think the restrictions were ineffectual; stories, especially romances of chivalry, managed to sneak through the net.

When I was a child, my family didn't attend any church regularly, but the stories from the Bible floated in the air of our lives, along with Roman and Greek myths: Jesus and the lepers, baby Moses in the basket in the river, Prometheus and fire. It did not matter whether the events in the stories actually happened or not, or whether the people had actually lived on the planet; what mattered was, like the stories in the novels read to me at night, that they were true (not literal — true).

My older brother, Kit, taught me to read when I was four, so I'd be ready, he said, for first grade. From then on I read books in trees, in old barns, on lawns, in backyards, on my mother's bed, in my own bed late at night. I could pick up anything I wanted. When a writer asked me what I was reading when I was twelve, I said, pompously, *The Rise and Fall of the Third Reich.*

When I was older, I found the great writers. I read Tolstoy's *Anna Karenina* and put it down and thought: How could he have done that? How did he know what a suicidal woman feels? How did he make me see and believe it? Later, when I wrote fiction, I saw that the lives of characters in a novel are partly the alternative lives the writer might have had and parts of the self (splintered, refracted, embellished): "Madame Bovary," said Flaubert, *"c'est moi."* I saw that in knowing them, *my characters,* I knew myself.

But now I could not read.

Part of the reason was the eye that had been "assaulted" (the right eye) tired very easily when I read with the left eye. (I could not actually read with the right eye; the letters were too distorted.) I felt it necessary to give the right eye a rest even though Dr. Lowe assured me it wasn't necessary. I felt it necessary. I wanted to "reverse" the visual field. I also wanted to preserve the "good" eye, not knowing what had caused the nerve inflammation in the "bad" eye. That eye, too, tired easily. I wore my not-rakish patch on my right eye when I worked, briefly, at the computer and when I, briefly, watched the evening news.

I had no morning newspaper, no novel to take to bed, nothing to read while eating lunch. That whole world was suddenly gone. I had no characters living inside me.

Then I remembered the audible books I had sent my mother when her eyes finally succumbed to macular degeneration; her pleasure at listening to her old favorites (*Rebecca, The Wind in the Willows*). I signed up at a Web site and downloaded *Middlemarch* to my laptop and, in the evening, lugged it to bed with my earphones. Vincent looked over at me and the laptop.

"Isn't that a little awkward?" he said.

"Yep," I said, "but it's fine."

What we didn't say was that I could not afford even a basic iPod because the doctor bills had begun to come in, and despite very good health insurance, the emergency room alone had wiped out my savings.

The next day I was lying on the window seat looking up at the Christmas tree, when Vincent walked in with a little white box and handed it to me.

I started to cry.

The envelope said, "N.G." Inside the card read, "Dearest N, Merry Christmas but mostly a help-you-take-care-of-your-eyes gift. Love, V." Inside the box was an iPod. It was silver. It was both light and heavy in my palm. I rushed to my study and transferred *Middlemarch* to it.

I lay down and listened to Dorothea's story, her girlish idealism, her painful lack of consciousness, her grim marriage to Mr. Casaubon, the cold, jealous, deeply alone Anglican minister, twenty years her senior. Casaubon, I thought — how I disliked him the first time I read the novel in my twenties; how much more sympathy I had for him now.

When I finished *Middlemarch,* I listened to Tolstoy's *The Death of Ivan Ilyich.* As Ivan Ilyich's friends gather at his funeral, one of them, hoping to get away soon to his club, thinks, "He must have done something terribly wrong . . . to have died." Then, in *War and Peace,* the doctors who come to treat Natasha Rostov prescribe different medicines almost every day and never talk to each other.

Doctors came to see her singly and in consultation, talked much in French, German, and Latin, blamed one another, and prescribed a great variety of medicines for all the diseases known to them, but the simple idea never occurred to any of them that they could not know the disease Natasha was suffering from, as no disease suffered by a live man can be known, for every living person has his own peculiarities and always has his own peculiar, personal, novel, complicated disease, unknown to medicine — not a disease of the lungs, liver, skin, heart, nerves, and so on mentioned in medical books, but a disease consisting of one of the innumerable combinations of the maladies of those organs.

The great writers spoke to my experience. They had found the words for my affliction and treated it with acerbic, bracing compassion. Tolstoy knew that doctors specialized in parts of the body and did not know how to look at it as a whole. He knew that people, fearing death, would try to blame death on the body in front of them. And the hope Tolstoy and Eliot offered was not tacked on, as an uplifting addendum, but was instead a satisfying resolution, born out of what it is to be human, out of deeply human hearts. They knew that we suffer and that each person's suffering is both singular and particular and also commonly held, universal. They did not turn away from it. They did not urge me to "think positively." (And Eliot, by creating Casaubon, gave me sympathy for that woman in Dr. Burks's office, in her bright clothes and perfect coiffure: what fear lay under her bromide?)

Tolstoy and Eliot had generosity, irony, and hope — three basic tools, it turned out, that I would need for survival in Oz.

CHAPTER 10

I began the round of specialists right before Christmas. At the urging of Dr. Lowe, I made an appointment with a neuro-ophthalmologist at UCLA. Vincent drove me down because neither of us felt that I could drive alone, and we knew they would dilate my eyes. I had never gone to a medical appointment with Vincent, never imagined this taking place. Now I saw myself following Vincent around from doctor to doctor with the same vague, worn expression I had seen on the woman in Dr. Lowe's waiting room.

My father had driven the back alleys of Las Cruces to avoid the police, as his driver's license had long expired, to get my mother's blood pressure medicine; Vincent's stepmother drove Vincent's father from Marin County into San Francisco for his lung doctor. Each day was planned around the doctors' appointments, until the appointments were all that was left. One spouse shouldered the other — the two-person partnership. This would be our fate, inevitably, I now understood. That I had never recognized this before, never imagined it, was part of my former life, in that other country, from which I was now separated by the glass wall. What had I imagined when I thought of us growing old? I had not. "Let's do this forever."

We took the coast highway. I watched the sea, gray and dark green in the winter light. At UCLA what caught my eye outside the Jules Stein Eye Institute were birds of paradise in huge planters and a man with a white cane. It was December 23, days before Christmas; the clinics were deserted. A solitary guard sat in a small office chair in an empty hall on the first floor. I remembered, as we went up in the elevator, that Jules Stein had been an impresario from Indiana who built a big band business into MCA.

Dr. Burks had said that I would have to pay attention to my symptoms because the tests were all negative. "We will have to rely on you," she said. I had made a list that would later fill notebooks: headache, stiffness in shoulders, temple pain, fatigue, weight loss. I brought a list of medications. Insurance card. And also a copy of a novel I wrote, without quite knowing why. When we got to the fifth floor, I went to the bathroom and in the mirror saw my cheeks fat and red from the steroids, the face of a bloated drunk. I turned away from my own reflection. I had been a reasonably nice-looking woman and was vain. Now my looks had disappeared in a matter of weeks. I thought of the women who lost their hair, my mother in her wig. I felt a deep fear in my stomach: Vincent would be repulsed by my looks. He would find someone else. In the months to come, Vincent's aunt, Malinda, who photographs everyone and carefully pastes them into albums, took no photos of me. I saw, later, how kind this was, how much she knew.

The waiting room was practically empty. I went to the reception desk, where the woman behind it ignored me. I cleared my throat. She went on working. I stood there hoping she was working on something important (resuscitation by typing?) until she, grumpy, asked me for my insurance card without looking up. I gave it to her, turned, and walked over to a worn but comfortable tan leather chair. On my new iPod, I listened to Alfred Brendel playing Schubert. I remembered watching him play his last, retirement concert at Carnegie Hall and how, as the ovations filled the hall again and again, he played again and again until his hands turned red.

A young, dark-haired woman called my name. Walking Vincent and me down the hall, she did not speak to either one of us. She ordered me to sit in a chair and dimmed the lights. When I told her I had a scar on the macula of my right eye and therefore needed to start the eye chart at a higher line than I would eventually be able to read, she ignored me. She tapped her pencil as I struggled with the chart. The sight in my right eye was 20/40 minus 1, the worst it had been in decades. She dumped us back in the waiting room without a word. Vincent read *The New York Times,* and I listened to Alfred, until another woman, older, nicer, placed us in an examining room.

A string of young residents, all of whom looked as if they would rather be anywhere but here (it was, after all, the holidays), did depth and color perception tests: Escher-like paintings with numbers hidden in dots of color and cartoon animals that popped up or did not. I had the dispiriting feeling of failing test after test. Like the blotches on the visual field, I saw what I had lost: I had lost color distinction in the right eye, I had lost almost all my ability to see red. Finally a young woman arranged herself in front of me, asked me to look at her nose, and held her long arms wide. She asked me to tell her the number of fingers she was holding up at the edge of my peripheral vision. This, I gathered, was the Jules Stein version of the visual field test. Vincent said later that she must have minored in modern dance.

They dilated my eyes. They numbed my eyes. They stuck the tip of a pen into the eyeball to take my pressure. Then they all trooped out, leaving me exhausted. Vincent immediately brought up the subject of what stoves I might want to replace our ancient one, then moved on to refrigerators and beds. Neither one of us had had the time to even look for replacements. Our icebox was freezing vegetables in their bin; our stove had to be turned up to 500 to roast potatoes. Then Dr. A, a tall man wearing a sagging suit, walked in. His eyes were intelligent and weary. The residents marched in behind him, like cadets on parade.

Dr. A asked me if I owned a cat. Had it scratched me? My cat doesn't scratch me, I said, and understood from his expression that this was more information than he

120

wanted. Red splotchy rash? He peered through the instrument at my eyes. He stood back and allowed the residents to take a look, one by one. Only one of them spoke to me. When the last of the six was ready, Dr. A touched my arm briefly, the only human contact I had, and said gently, "Just one more."

Finally he stood back. Vincent had been taking notes and was ready with his pen.

"I am fifty-fifty," he said, "inflammatory or circulatory. I can't tell which. The nerve is no longer inflamed."

"What leads you toward circulatory?" I asked.

"The pattern of the visual loss," he replied. "The MRI."

Then he stopped and looked away. I stopped, too, though I had more questions. The specialist's time allotment, I would learn, is ten minutes. After that you are no longer a model patient. He wanted me to repeat the blood tests I had had when I first was diagnosed with uveitis, all of them. Send the results to him; he would send me his report in January.

I found myself thanking him profusely. After he left, I asked his nurse to give him the copy of my novel I had brought along.

When I called his office to ask for a

follow-up appointment, I was told by a cross receptionist that Dr. A did not do follow-ups; he only did diagnoses. I never saw him again. This is common among specialists, as it turns out — the one visit, the "diagnosis" or lack of one, no follow-up, and the vague, noncommittal "report." (According to *The New York Times,* specialists now outnumber internists two to one.)

I had had faith in Dr. A. I thought he would figure out the problem; that was the role, I thought, of a medical specialist. I thought he would marshal his considerable resources and solve it. But that piece of faith would soon vanish, for me and for Vincent. Several months later, when a friend asked Vincent how things were going, he replied, "She has an appointment with another useless world-renowned specialist."

We walked out into the clear winter twilight in Los Angeles and down the parking ramp. We had been there three and a half hours. As we passed the birds of paradise, I felt a sense of being robbed of something.

It would take me a long time, almost two years, to figure out what it was. What kept returning to my mind was giving my novel to the nurse. Why had I done that?

As we got in the car, Vincent said, "Do you have to go through *that* every time?"

"What?" I asked.

He looked at me with concern: "What they did to you," he said. "The eye chart, the dilation, the numbing, the pencil in the eye, those weird colored tests, the residents . . ."

"I haven't seen an eye specialist in a while," I said. "But yes, that's the drill." I thought to myself: Why is it the drill? Not so much the eye chart and tests, but the attitude and the numbers of people. The feeling of being a thing to test, not a person to heal.

I asked that question of a friend who is a doctor a few weeks later, and he replied, "Teaching hospitals are set up for the students, not for the patients."

We drove home to a little trattoria Vincent had wanted to try — the first new restaurant I'd been in since early December — and split a giant, expensive rib eye. The room was brightly lit and full of people, and I felt as if I were living inside a kaleidoscope with my dilated eyes and steroid-filled brain. Vincent reached his hand across the table.

Three and half weeks after "it," I had no diagnosis. The nerve was actually not back to normal (an MRI would confirm that) but was not noticeably inflamed. I was taking

60 milligrams of prednisone a day. The temporal artery biopsy (for autoimmune inflammation in the arteries) was negative.

Like other people who live a middle-class professional life, I had thought that I could manage to control or contain or overcome almost anything. I had known this so completely that I had not actually consciously thought it out. And because I have been a working journalist, I knew the power of connection. The person with the power over any given situation, the person with the information needed for the story, was only three degrees of separation, if that, away.

I had tracked down the people who harbored Patty Hearst when she was on the lam, by sitting on a doorstep in San Francisco for three days. I had convinced a juror from the Dan White trial after their verdict to talk to me. (Dan White assassinated George Moscone and Harvey Milk in 1978.) I had talked my way past police barricades and through rioters burning police cars. I knew my way around.

I had found that studio in the Village; a friend knew a friend. At that time I had marveled at how easy it was, how small the circle. I had not fully understood that the circle was small because the circle of educated professionals is small. I had not considered what it was to not have these connections or any way of breaking in. To be, in a word, powerless.

Outside my close circle of friends and family, people seemed to believe that my medical situation could be managed, that all it lacked was information, that what I needed was . . .

"You should find . . ."

"Have you tried . . . ?"

"How about . . . ?"

Hanging up from their well-meaning phone calls, I would feel more isolated, more inside the glass wall than I had before we talked. They were trying to *manage the situation*. Things don't happen out of nowhere. They have a cause. They have effects.

Their response was complicated by the lack of general knowledge regarding autoimmune disorders, not to mention lack of medical knowledge. Autoimmune disease, as Bevra Hahn, the head of rheumatology at UCLA, would later explain to me, is a situation in which the immune system — or antibodies — attacks the body's own tissue.

In the medical literature, there is an almost literary term for it: "the failure of self-tolerance."

Dr. Hahn's research has led her to believe that autoimmunity is a disease of civilization. "The cavemen's immune system was set on a hair trigger to attack infections, and they were exposed to infections every minute. But we are 'too clean.' We are not exposed to infections, especially as children, but we have the same immune system, which is looking for trouble. In autoimmune disorders, the antibodies are in overload; their regulation is wrong." She went on to say that each of the immune diseases has a genetic component: the genetic predisposition appears, she said, to be contained in the target tissue. Each autoimmune disease — MS, lupus, rheumatoid arthritis — has its own bag of tricks. A friend who has MS put it perfectly: "You never know who is going to be in the guest house tonight."

Each disease has its own trigger, its own genetic history, and possibly its own code. It has taken Dr. Hahn's medical lifetime (she just retired at seventy-three) to begin to grasp lupus.

Despite this complexity, the popular culture responds to mysterious illness as if the victim's personality had caused it. Diseases that have no discernible cause are the most obvious choices. Susan Sontag wrote about this twenty years ago in her revelatory book *Illness as Metaphor,* when there was an actual phrase — "the cancer personality." Before cancer, the disease was TB. "Sensitive" people — poets, artists — got TB. Once the bacillus that causes TB was found, that link faded. Now the new diseases vulnerable to the "personality" cause are autoimmune.

We want to have answers, we want to explain how things happen, we want cause and effect. Autoimmune diseases are caused by as-yet-unknown factors that will, in time, be known. But we have so little tolerance for not knowing, for reaching the limits of reason, that we make up stories that will explain, satisfy, put it to bed.

Shortly after I saw Dr. A, I talked to a friend on the East Coast. I knew him fairly well and had told him years before that my mother's mother, elderly and alone, grieving the sudden loss of her beloved husband, had taken an overdose of sleeping pills.

The morning he asked me what was going on with me, I told him an autoimmune disorder. He gave it some thought, asked me more questions, and then said, "Your grandmother committed suicide, didn't she? We could think of autoimmune as a form of suicide."

I did not know what to say. I didn't know how to get off the line. He wanted an explanation that would . . . would what? I asked myself as I put down the phone.

My thoughts went back to that first day, when I crossed the street from Dr. Lowe to Dr. Burks. I thought about the doctors and the boys on the street who had sailed past me, and the wall that fell between us.

I had thought that the wall appeared because I felt so suddenly ill, so entirely different from how I had felt hours before. I had thought the wall was my own work, but now I understood that it was also theirs. The people on the street that day, the men and women who called and gave me advice, the man who likened an autoimmune disorder to suicide were not only not living where I was, they were determined to hold fast against the knowledge that such a place existed, outside cause and effect. *It must be because my grandmother committed suicide. He must have done something terribly wrong. It must be something he ate or drank or did.* Or else? I finally understood. Or else it could happen to them.

My close friends, I saw later, were trying very hard to figure out what to do. They were climbing that hill of sand I had climbed when Jodie's Frank died. I didn't fit into easy categories. I didn't have the flu, for which short-term chicken soup and phone calls would have done; I didn't (or so they thought) have cancer, for which friends would have to put their own lives, and their own disasters, on hold. I had *something else.*

I was not giving them many clues. I had no experience with being vulnerable, in need. I did not want to be *beholden.* I feared self-pity. When I said something about feeling behind this wall, alone, to my friend Cynthia, she burst into tears. "That I can't reach you is not for lack of trying!"

The people who had encountered Oz themselves were the most confident. A friend who had almost died in a traffic accident when she was eighteen drove me to an exercise class twice a week so I could keep doing something. She was *there,* a dependable driver, giving hours out of her days. Another woman delivered a special tea to my doorstep every few weeks without knocking or asking to come in. When I finally saw her, she told me that she was operating under a tit-for-tat protocol: when she was undergoing chemo for breast cancer, I had delivered food to her door, and she had asked me to come inside to shave her head.

"I'll do the same, if you need it. Or rather" — she laughed ruefully — "some version of it."

A man from Trinity, who had serious cataracts in both eyes and macular degeneration, made dinner for us, leaving it on the porch with brief, factual notes.

I ran into another woman from church at the farmer's market, where I had moved over to the side of an aisle to avoid the crowds ravenous for winter squash. Margaret had stomach cancer. We nodded to each other. She stopped beside me.

"Do you," Margaret said, "tell people the truth when they ask how you are doing?"

I laughed. "Never. I don't want to watch their eyes glaze over."

A friend who had survived a blood disorder went with me to several appointments in Los Angeles, sitting in the ubiquitous waiting room, just to keep me company. Another (head concussion) drove down from the Bay Area to stay with me when Vincent had to travel. These people offered no sympathy, gave no advice, used no vacuous expressions. They did not tell me to think positively. Even the churchgoers never, ever mentioned "God." (The clichés that are possible when you use the word *God* are infinite.) In Oz, all that had been stripped away. But the people were not at a loss for words. They chose words that were spare, precise, laced with dark humor, *real*.

There were no long-lasting prescriptives. Debbie, from Houston, an American Baptist, left a voice message: "I am keeping you in my prayers. Not that that is going to make you better, but I certainly hope it's of some help."

I felt with them as if we were holding each other up in a tenuous circle, arms around each other. We were making it up as we went along.

About a week into the New Year, which had passed unnoticed — everything was now dated from December 1, 2009 — I was at the gym for the first time since "it," attempting to exercise, afraid to be on an elliptical trainer for fear of jolting the eye and thus was on a treadmill just walking dully along. I had situated myself next to a window so I could see a tree, a magnolia, which I watched rather than the TV. The world was what I wanted to see. The magnolia had large polished leaves and those huge, almost false white waxen blossoms. I was looking at the tree when something caught my eye, *caught my eye,* beneath it. It was a person, walking up the steps at the base of the tree to a low wall, where she sat down. She was talking, or her mouth was moving. A tall man followed her, but she seemed not to be

131

talking to him but rather to herself. He was watching her carefully. From the way he was attentive to her, his head cocked toward her, the distance between them (not too close but not too far), I figured he knew her. Was she talking to him? I could not tell. Her clothes were shabby: a red sweatshirt over a shapeless black skirt. Leggings. Gray running shoes. The layers of a homeless person, the body as a suitcase. I watched them off and on until they both got on a bus.

One night I watched a youngish couple walk in the door of our favorite Italian restaurant. We were sitting in the middle of the room, having requested a table near the window where we always sit, and having been told that the table where we always sit was reserved. I had been irritated by this. The couple came in the door, and my eye rested on them. She was holding tight to his arm, and her head was tilted at an odd angle — I realized finally that she could not see out of the center of her eyes but was trying to see out of the periphery. She could not have been more than forty. He was careful, but not condescending, as he led her to the table, our table, by the window. When they were seated, he moved his chair so he was sitting beside rather than across from her and led her through the menu.

I touched Vincent's arm.

He said, "If we couldn't have the table because of them, that's okay."

"Always," I said.

In a new ophthalmologist's waiting room, I watched a tired woman with a cane and a worried frown walking in. My eye caught her before I realized she was a woman I knew, a local judge and an Episcopal priest, who had been diagnosed, at just about the same time my affliction befell me, with stage-four melanoma.

I did not want to let her know I was there. I did not want to talk to her. I did not want to be that close to the thing that hovered over her. But I knew just before it happened that the nurse would call my name, and I'd be exposed. She did, and Colleen looked up. I walked over to her and said, "When this is over, may I join you?" and she said yes. Her eyes looked weary, as if she were looking at something over my shoulder. She smiled. When I came back, I sat down next to her and rather than feeling awkward, rather than worrying about what to say, I felt my way along what was, now, a familiar rope. Her disaster was much bigger than mine, her country far away, but we had things in common. We talked in low voices about the endless waiting rooms, the doctors, the protocols, the search. She had found a doctor she liked in San Diego finally, who had gotten her into a new trial, the fourth she had tried, and it seemed to be working. The tumors were shrinking. But she and her husband were working on the "bucket list." They would soon travel to London, just to see it again.

Finally I understood that my eyes were going to the vulnerable, the sick, the homeless first now, whereas before I had seen them last. I would say my eyes *rested* on them now, whereas in the past my eyes *passed over* them. I gradually came to *see* that I had been, in my busy, travel-filled life, very much like Ivan Ilyich's friends, and the people who called me offering advice. I — busy, athletic, healthy — was not like the others, the ones who were sick. *It,* whatever *it* was, would not happen to me.

I was big, unlike them, who were small. I had connections. I had somewhere to get to.

Now the connections, the power, the places to get to were straws in the wind. I was small. My eye was going to the vulnerable, the small, the people who were like me. The last ones were now first.

A woman at church made me a prayer

shawl. These shawls were hand-knitted from acrylic yarn so you could wash them, then blessed by those who were part of this "ministry." I had seen them, piled up on the welcome table at the coffee hour in strange bright colors, and cringed. But then Betty Bickel told me she had made me one. Betty had managed to be the stereotype of a churchgoing regular — elderly, quiet, dutiful — but I knew her to be instead courageous, original, and kind. She also makes the best lemon bars. When she told me she had made me a shawl, I practically ran down to church to pick it up. It was blue acrylic. I brought it home and lay down beside it. Junior jumped up on the bed and headed for it. I held on to it with one hand the way children hold their blankie. We both fell asleep. When Vincent came home, he looked at it with some concern. "Betty Bickel made it," I said. "Oh," he said, "then it's fine." After that we called it, one word: bettybikelsprayershawl.

"I think it works," I told Betty when I thanked her.

And she looked at me as if to say *Duh*.

I held on to the prayer shawl as I lay awake in the dark. I thought about the woman under the window at the gym. And then I remembered the story of the blind beggar in various gospels. It is one of those simple, direct stories in the Bible: a man blind from birth begs in Bethsaida. Jesus of Nazareth passes through and, seeing him, takes him by the hand and leads him to the fields surrounding the village, away from the prying eyes of the religious authorities. There Jesus kneels down in the dust and makes a paste out of dirt and his own spit and smoothes it over the blind man's eyes.

I had been drawn to the story before I feared losing my sight. I had liked its detail (taking him by the hand, away from the village elders) and the use of those rough materials — dust and spit. And what the man is recorded as seeing is reminiscent of what Oliver Sacks reported people who are blind from birth to see when they are operated on to remove cataracts.

"What do you see?" his friends ask him.

He replies, "I see men as trees, walking."

The story felt true.

In the night alone, pondering the story, my interest oddly was not in the "miracle" part. Instead I thought about what it would be like to have a doctor lead you by the hand and get down on his knees. What I thought about in the dark was the fellowship, that old word, of Jesus. Extending his hand and leading this man, unable to see where he was going. At the time of Jesus, illness was thought to be caused by sin: either one's own or one's parent's sin. (The "cancer personality" is not far from this first-century cause/effect.) So to heal someone was more than personal; it broke through a code, a social ostracism.

Jesus led the blind man out to the fields, away from prying, judging, powerful eyes. And there he knelt down.

Then, I thought in the night, is this the eye that sees?

■ ■ ■ ■

PART TWO:
LIMBO

■ ■ ■ ■

CHAPTER 11

Vincent and I decided not to use certain metaphors. *Blind drunk. Blind as a bat. We don't see eye to eye.* We used *deaf as a bat,* until I started to lose my hearing. I made lists of what to ask the doctors, of what I needed to know.

On the last day of December, Dr. Burks ordered a full-body CT scan. Sometimes, she said, tumors can cause these weird aberrations. In a closetlike room I removed my clothes and "everything metal," put on a blue-and-white-dotted cotton gown, and presented myself to the clothed technicians. I lay down on the narrow white bed. The nurse and technician left the room and talked to me through a microphone in the machine.

"Take a breath. Hold it. Now breathe out." The cot passed me through a large white doughnut. I closed my eyes. It made a noise between a whirr and a buzz.

The scan report came back. The radiologist noted "emphysema" scarring. He noted a 1.4-centimeter "nodule" in the upper area of my left lung.

Dr. Mesipam told me I needed to see a lung specialist. I went to see Dr. Robert Wright. His office, like Dr. Burks's, was just around the corner from our house. He was tall with prematurely white hair, he had an accent that carried a trace of his English Montreal boyhood, and he loved wilderness. We bonded over Patagonia.

He assured me that I did not have emphysema and was the first to explain to me that radiologists tend to go overboard in their notes. The nodule, he said after a brief hesitation, was not cancer, but they would have to "follow it."

"I smoked, you know," I said.

"Yes," he said. "For how long? And when did you quit?"

I asked him why he thought it wasn't cancer, and he shrugged and hesitated: "Forty years of practice."

Much of me believed him. I quit smoking twenty-five years ago — surely my odds were good. But now cancer, which had not been part of the drumbeat of worry, joined it. On the Internet, I noted, lesions in the lung caught below 10 centimeters increased the survival rate by nine years. Above that, the rates fell to four months.

I had been, at first, greedy for the Internet, typing in "optic nerve inflammation" with steady hands. But I learned my lesson fast. "May cause a complete or partial loss of vision." "MS is a known cause." The various horrible possibilities just made things worse. My imagination did just fine on its own. On the other hand, with no diagnosis, I found certain, unhysterical Web sites: Uptodate, for clinicians; the Mayo Clinic; Physicians' First Watch. I checked them when new information came in. On these sites, I found a couple of possibilities, rare disorders that cause trouble in the optic nerve and are sometimes related to uveitis: systemic lupus, neuro-sarcoidosis, Lyme disease. I wrote down their names.

Dr. Mesipam, my internist, said, "It's not cancer." I looked over his shoulder at the locust tree outside his window. "I'm going to have to believe you," I said. He was wearing one of the French shirts his wife buys for him in a deep violet that set off his dark skin. It was perfectly ironed, the creases like neat incisions. Dr. Mesipam's offices are in Montecito, a wealthy forested town just south of Santa Barbara. (Oprah keeps a house there.) When he first started practicing and was looking for an office, colleagues warned him that "those people" would not see a doctor who had a foreign name (Babji Mesipam) and almost-black skin. Now he is a doctor to celebrities; people battle to get in to see him. I once had to crawl over Jonathan Winters's knees to get to an examining room. Dr. Mesipam views this situation with permanent irony.

I told him about my visit to Dr. A and said I had another appointment in L.A., to see a specialist in uveitis, in early January.

"Do I have to go back to L.A.?" I whined.

He looked at me and said, "You may need to go to L.A. dozens of times. As often as it takes." And then with a hint of exasperation, "I would go to L.A. very often if it were me. It's your eyes."

I had a rather large speaking engagement coming up in February, I told him.

"Where?" he said.

"Virginia," I said.

"Let's see," he said. "That's at least three planes."

I counted. "At least."

"I am going to have to say that it's better not to do that," he said. "We don't know what we're dealing with. I am going to ground you until May."

I postponed Virginia. A talk in Louisville. Then another and another. I felt a combination of anxiety, fear, and relief. Anxiety at the loss of income, fear that I would fall off the radar of the lecture circuit, and relief that I did not have to pack those bags, print out those boarding passes, check into the ubiquitous hotels. My world shrank. I had nowhere to get to.

Then suddenly, I stopped going to church. At first it was because I could not be around crowds of any size. I was still worn out. My sight was not stable. From the way people looked at me, I was obviously sick. I was walking into the church office one day to pick up bettybickelsprayershawl, when another parishioner, a woman I knew slightly, was coming out. She seemed momentarily shocked, then rearranged her expression just enough to present a bland, distant, pained expression and asked in a lowered tone: "How *are* you?" It was, God forbid, *sympathy.* Her look said: *Oh, I am so sorry you are* over there, *helpless. Unlike me, who is not.* I knew the look: I had once handed it out freely to people in wheelchairs, to homeless men on the street, to women with bald heads. Now it was handed to me.

I knew from working as a prayer minister at Trinity that many people there had drowned. Prayer ministers work in teams of two. During communion, we stand at the back of the church near the baptismal font and wait. When a person approaches us, we stand with our arms around each other, enclosing a small, separate piece of air. (It was this circle — people holding each other up — that I remembered when people who had been sick themselves helped me out.)

The man or woman would then let us know the truth about his or her life: the daughter starving herself; the lymphoma out of control; the husband who may have embezzled. The prayer ministers took turns praying out loud, which was always just about what came into our heads. I was almost always surprised at what came out of my mouth or the mouth of the person standing next to me, the words that seemed to come from the best place in us and also from another place, an otherness. The words were not sentimental or necessarily "religious"; they were words dug up on the spot, and they tended to have a fresh, original scent. Then one of us would take out a little sterling silver box containing oil on cotton and anoint the person's forehead. After all that, the same person would march back to the pew.

The trick to keeping a confidence is to keep it secret not only from others but from the self, so I would see the same people after we had prayed together and not quite remember what they had told me. I felt as if I had left their secrets either in the air back by the baptismal font or in the font itself, which seemed to be the best place for them. But several times, more often than not, when I saw one of them holding a mug of coffee or eating a homemade cookie at the coffee hour, we would exchange a look across the space and the people between us. In that look was an acknowledgment of the disaster that had happened to them.

The irony was that in this place where you could cry in a pew or go to a prayer minister to pray, it was still hard to be actually sick, actually vulnerable. The very same woman who had told me of her lymphoma stood at the coffee hour trying to look upright and purposeful. The prayer ministers and the priests knew how many people were suffering; the rest of us did not.

I was embarrassed to be sick; I felt I had failed in some fundamental way.

On a Sunday in early January, after the news from Dr. Mesipam that I would not be traveling, I made my way back to a service on Sunday. I sat at the back of the church, in a pew that was in shadow, and leaned against the plastered stone wall. I stood up for the opening hymn. With one eye, I read the opening prayer along with everyone else. I sang a hymn. I listened to a decent sermon. Something wasn't quite right. I felt a gap open up between me and the service, between my suffering body and the words I had repeated over and over for forty years. In *The New York Times,* Samuel Freedman wrote about a woman who had been raped and her first Sunday back in church. In the state she was in, the service did not console her. It had an "empty predictability." That summed it up for me. I could not find a place in the service that gave me comfort or a place where I could expose my vulnerability.

And when it was time to say the creed, I stood up with the crowd. When they said, "I believe in God the Father Almighty," nothing came out of my mouth. They made their way through "Jesus his only Son," "Born of the Virgin Mary," "Ascended into Heaven and is seated at the right hand of God."

I stood there mute, and when everyone else said, "Amen," I sat down.

The words were suddenly *all wrong.* It was not so much about concepts or theology.

They were wrong *for me.* For where I was. I was so small. I was so scared. One might think a God that was Almighty would have been good news. But He was not. All these people — the Father, the Son, the Virgin — in that formal declaration were very far away, in another country. Not in my country. Not in Oz.

It's easy to imagine that I was angry at that Almighty God because He had let me fall sick, but at that moment, at least, that wasn't what I felt. I felt . . . alone. I remembered all the people who had come to us prayer ministers and told stories of pain, anguish, and illness, and then stood upright in their pews, and at the coffee hour. How had we gotten to the place where the man who took the blind man by the hand was nowhere in sight?

And the words *almighty, holy, virgin, only* weren't any help at all. I had said them, with more and more reluctance over the years, but the scalding power of illness had swept away pretense.

The word *heretic* came to my mind; a word based on the Greek for "choice."

I walked out the door into a cold January day and did not go back.

I told no one. I had enough guilt left over from . . . where? The ether? That if I didn't

149

go to church on Sunday, it was my fault.

The church secretary asked me a week or so later if I wanted my name on the weekly prayer list, and I said yes, please. I was grateful for the thought that someone might pray for me, whatever that meant to them, and grateful for the prayer shawl and for the people who, trained from years of church, had brought dinners to us. I was grateful for the building and for Mark and for the hundreds of people at Trinity and for the effort that the larger church had made at keeping alive deeper meanings. But it was not a place I could be.

Years ago, on a Sunday morning, my friend Ann Jaqua picked me up for church. She came in while I downed the last cup of tea, and there was Vincent sitting at the dining room table reading *The New York Times.* He greeted her, offered her a seat. She declined and said, "I don't know if I have wanted to have this picture in my mind of the alternative to going to church."

The Sunday after I didn't say the creed, rather than take a shower and rush out the door for the ten o'clock service, I sat with Vincent and read the *Times.*

He noticed, of course. Finally, on the third Sunday, he asked. I said I was taking a break.

"It means so much to you," my agnostic husband said with a worried frown.

"I know," I said. "I can't explain it right now."

After a couple of Sundays — by this time the wild luxury of sitting around in my sweats reading the Style Section had started to get old — I realized that there was something that had been hidden under *going to church.* Something raw.

In January in the rain, I ran in front of an SUV to try to save a dog.

We had been walking with friends on the bluffs above the beach. They were driving up from L.A., on their way to the Bay Area. As we drove back to our house for dinner, in a two-car caravan, we saw a dog weaving between cars on the narrow road to the beach. We pulled over. We stopped. It was twilight. Our friend Patrick remembers thinking, "This is the kind of situation where people get hurt."

He and I got out of our respective cars. Just as I stood on the edge of the road, the dog, crouching on the other side, stood up. I screamed "No!" and ran toward him. I heard the screech of brakes. I saw the lights. "This close," Vincent said later, holding his fingers an inch apart.

I was so terrified of what I had done that I kept reliving it, then forcing it out of my mind.

At that point I knew that the steroids had affected my brain.

"My father became very chatty on steroids," my friend Martha said. I was very chatty.

I was in it. It had me.

I could drive, after practicing in the neighborhood. I drove more slowly and did not take the right periphery for granted. A new Whole Foods Market opened near our house, and I drove over to check it out. I was soothed by the 1960s music, by the bins of food, by the cheeses laid out to taste under plastic domes. I held on to the cart as if it were a walker and wandered around. I took to shopping two or three times a week — pretending to shop, that is, just to feel soothed by the music and the cartons of food. *The world goes forward,* I wrote in my journal. *I do not.*

One of my friends wrote to me that she and her husband were going to Italy. Another casually mentioned a week in New York. It didn't even have to be Rome or New York. They spoke of going out to movies during the week, staying out late at restaurants, working on the weekends, doing a "bunch" of errands. They had so much *energy*. Their lives were so bizzy. *They had somewhere to get to.* My friends could not have known it, but for me what they were doing was . . . out of reach . . . way over *there*.

One day, as I was driving to Whole Foods for my biweekly vacation, I found my usual route blocked. Signs were up that the road would be closed intermittently for four months. A backhoe was positioned in the creek bed under the bridge I usually drove over. Later I walked to the park that the creek ran through and read the signs that said the creek restoration was now in full progress, as part of a larger project to help bring back steelhead trout to southern California. The backhoe was taking out the concrete that the Army Corps of Engineers had put in there in the 1940s to "prevent" floods. I had of course seen this creek many times in the twenty years we had lived near it. The concrete along its edges made it odd and unattractive. It always had bits of trash, plastic bags mainly, somewhere in its waters. It went dry in the summer, as do many of Southern California's creeks, and then it was an alleyway in the city; people crossed it if they couldn't figure out another way of getting from one side of the park to the other and dropped trash on the way. I didn't have a whole lot of hope for this restoration, but I watched its progress. I waited.

I had a new job, in addition to my half-time job at Patagonia and my half-time job as a writer — managing my care. I had four doctors in town: Dr. Mesipam, Dr. Burks, Dr. Lowe, and Dr. Wright. I had seen Dr. A the neuro-ophthalmologist. I now had to go back to Los Angeles to see Dr. Narsing Rao, a specialist in uveitis, one of three top specialists in the world, at the Doheny Eye Institute. Dr. Rao had seen me every few months for several years after the first episode of uveitis. Like many specialists, he was in his clinic only once a week. The rest of the time he traveled, gave lectures, attended worldwide conferences. He was bizzy.

The receptionist told me that Dr. Rao had one morning appointment at ten o'clock on a Tuesday. Getting from Santa Barbara to downtown Los Angeles in a car during the week in the midmorning is impossible. I knew this. I weighed staying with a friend in Los Angeles the night before but was reluctant to leave my own bed. I weighed leaving at five a.m. and having breakfast somewhere nearby. I weighed simply sitting in traffic for four hours. I could leave at six. Then I remembered that my eyes would be dilated, and so I could not drive alone. Vincent had a day at work that he could not cancel. My friends had done so much; how could I ask them to sit in a doctor's waiting room in Los Angeles?

It was the beginning of not only managing my medical care (that is, balancing the doctors, reporting to each one what the other had said, keeping notes, and remembering to bring scans, lists of medications, blood tests to each visit) but also managing when the appointments would take place and how many there would be and how I would get to them. It's what all patients of my category undertake.

Then I realized there was a train to Los Angeles. In the West, unlike the East, we do not regard trains as actual transportation, because they aren't scheduled to run when people want to travel and they are rarely on time. When I looked it up, however, I saw that the Surfliner left at six forty-five in the morning and got into L.A. two and a half hours later. I could take a cab from the station to the medical center. Later I would discover a free shuttle bus.

That morning I rose at five, dressed, and had breakfast. Vincent took me to the station. He told me to sit on the right side so that I could see the ocean. About fifteen minutes later I got on the train.

I watched the ocean waves that seemed to be right beneath the tracks, the beaches, the coves. Near Patagonia headquarters, I saw ducks floating on the Ventura River, where it meets the sea. I saw, inland, a brown rabbit sitting still in the sun. A black horse with its head in a feed bin that hung off a fence; a crow lifting off a pile of garbage underneath oak trees.

Yellow rocks in Chatsworth Park and Stoney Point, where Vincent's uncle had climbed as a boy to hawks' nests and where I had climbed with the Honettes.

To be where I am but to wait.

A small ranch, with trucks, corrals, a circle for exercising horses, a soothing anachronism in the midst of the sprawl of the suburbs of Los Angeles.

Mountains in the distance, the coast range. Three tunnels following one another. The total dark of a tunnel.

The smell of a skunk

Why is the information in the present needed? Where does it come from? Why did I think this?

Faceless gray brick warehouses with circular fire escapes from the roof.
Costco.
A man running for his car.
I want something to make me feel content (safe, unafraid) all the time, thus drugs. Thus what has come to mean religion.
An electrical power plant with many tall power poles.
Tumbleweeds.
Metal low warehouses with lots of graffiti/tags.
Tumbleweeds.
Swimming pools in backyards, some oval, some kidney-shaped, the blue water inviting, alternating with horse corrals.
Trains are the only way to see people's backyards.
A horse trail running along the railroad tracks on which I would see, on later train rides, a man who looked like a real cowboy.
Planes at a large private airport.
Dust.
Locust trees with purple flowers.
Three men wearing white chef's hats coming out of a door.
An ambulance in a car lot.
Palms.
A woman in a golf cart.
A concrete water channel with algae at the

bottom.

Businesses of the same genre congregate.

In Van Nuys, busted car country: used lots followed by smashed lots. A front end with the hood in the windshield.

I wonder who managed to survive these wrecks.

"We'll see your sedan and raise you a Passat" on a billboard.

A woman looks at herself in the train window as she gets off the train in Burbank. Self-storage.

Another channel. *Were these channels creeks or rivers?*

Stacks of shipping pallets.

Right beside the tracks, a trailer with a neat awning, a picnic table, and cords of stacked firewood. A man standing beside the trailer cooking breakfast on a grill, as in Nicaragua, or Mexico.

A burst of human life.

The "Déjà Vu" bar advertises pole dancers.

Broken school buses.

A flock of pigeons rising.

Palm trees in containers.

A pile of paint cans.

Rows of clothes on racks.

The warehouses get spiffier as we near L.A.

"Import" and "export."

A bakery.

Trucks with tanks of oxygen.

Janitorial supply.

A wide green lawn that turns out to be a cemetery.

Bob Hope Airport.

A bald man in a red shirt, pacing.

Fryes Electronics with its signature: a life-size flying saucer crashed into its sign.

Garbage out on streets in a neighborhood.

Rose bougainvillaea spreading over a wall.

Two police cars in a wrecking yard. *Which makes me smile, involuntarily: my old "pig" feelings from the sixties still there.*

Stacks of broken things in big plastic crates.

Dump trucks (which I wrote as "dumb" trucks).

"Central Casting."

"Gold'n West," another strip club.

The strippers: where do they come from?

A tin shed.

Trees, a relief to the eye.

A brick warehouse.

I wonder whether inside the many warehouses are sweatshops.

More shipping pallets.

What is shipped? Where?

An American flag poking out of a small yard.

Driving through New England after 9/11: bunting on the fire stations.

A jasmine vine.
Buckets.
Razor wire. *Always, razor wire.*
Two cypress trees.
A blue tin shed.
A red tin shed
A yellow tin shed.
I can still see.
Galilee Mission Center.
Plumbing supply next to another strip club.
A small billboard: "Share curiosity, read together."
An RV with a blue ocean painted on its side.
I'd like to hop in.
A field with crows.
Fir trees along a fence.
A turquoise wall.
A little cottage, alone in the midst of the parking lots and warehouses.
Does someone live there?
Another unpaved lot with large palm trees, and tags.
Vines covering an old awning factory, long gone.
"People should respect each other" written on a sheet and hung off a roof.
A mural of faces in glowing colors.
An empty lot with tires.
Plastic covers a mound of dirt.
Then, suddenly, the part of the Los Angeles

River that has been allowed to return to its wild state from a channel. Grass and cottonwoods along the sand and clay banks. It had surged recently, lots of debris on the shore. Rocks in the middle. Birds floating. *A feeling, like the man cooking breakfast near his trailer, unorganized, free.*
Trees trees trees.
Small yellow square things.
Empty dirt lots — with pieces of paving.
The train is slowing.
A bamboo screen on the stairwell of neat subsidized housing apartments next to the tracks.
Bottomless freight cars.
"Low low prices."
Store-it-all.
Worlds disappearing, worlds colliding.
Union Station.

It was much easier to stay in the present while sitting on a train. The train moves, the present changes.

Each thing I had seen had information in it; each one either mirrored our troubled lives or was their antidote. And the attention I had paid to each of the things — a pole dancer lounge, a man who sold wood by the tracks — gave me what amounted to a particle of time. Those particles, rather

161

than disappearing from me in inattention, now remained. I still see them.

The Doheny Eye Institute was on the University of Southern California medical campus, at the edge of downtown L.A. near the Five freeway. The retinal center and the neuro-ophthalmology center shared the fourth floor.

In the waiting room were rows of comfortably upholstered chairs and a long row of windows. A man wearing bandages on his eyes was in a wheelchair next to a woman who was holding his hand. People were not reading magazines or watching TV. Or working on laptops. They were mainly staring into the space in front of them.

A polite young woman measured my sight. It had improved slightly from December. I felt a flood of relief. She dilated my eyes. She numbed them and took their pressures. She led me to another part of the floor, where a doctor shot dye into my veins and a young woman from Austria with a Spanish accent took fluoresceins. She measured the thickness of my retina with what is called an OCT. "Please try not to blink," she said. Then she led me back to Dr. Rao's section.

Dr. Rao's fellow, Dr. J, took my "history."

He was tall and brash. He took what looked like haphazard notes. He would then report to Dr. Rao what he had heard me tell him, the bizarre system of "telephone" common in specialists' clinics.

Dr. Rao was ten years older than the last time I had seen him, when he had told me to take vitamin E, a year before studies showed the vitamin improved circulation. Ophthalmology is one of the hardest of the medical fields, gathering the most intelligent and patient medical students usually at the very top of their classes. To then be at the top of the specialist field is to be very bright indeed and to be very patient. Dr. Rao is also warm and genial, born in India. When I first saw him, in the 1980s, I would list his name on other doctors' medical information sheets under: "Your Doctors." Very often a nurse or receptionist would mispronounce his name and then come very close to a snigger.

Dr. Rao greeted me in his round cheerful voice. I could glimpse, as the sleeves of his white coat drew back when he shook my hand, a beautiful Italian suit. I once walked past three of Dr. Rao's white coats hanging off hangers, fresh from the laundry, and I felt as if the coats were him. He asked politely if he might look at my eyes.

"Hum," he said as he looked through the glass. I remembered his voice from a decade ago, its soft human sound.

"The nerve is not inflamed now," he said. "I do not immediately know what caused it. The uveitis — I wonder if it worked backward, along the nerve?" He sat with his hands in his lap looking at me. The retina was healthy, he said.

"What about the visual field?" I asked.

He said they would take that later, here, but from the reports I had sent him, it looked as if things were stable. Dr. Burks had said the visual field was about the only thing they had, it seemed to her, to measure how things were going.

"What about MS?" I asked.

"I don't think so," he said. "But you should have an MRI." He suggested I see one of his colleagues, Dr. Q, a neuro-ophthalmologist, and he asked one of his nurses to call him.

Dr. Rao suggested I start tapering the prednisone. I was just getting ready to beg him to see me again, having experienced Dr. A's "no follow-up," when he said, "Please make an appointment for two months from now." As he said good-bye to me, he held my arm.

Dr. J came back into the room after Dr. Rao had left.

Thinking of him as friendly and knowledgeable, I asked, "Is it possible that I have something called neuro-sarcoidosis?"

"You are like my mother," he said. "You are looking things up on the Internet. No, it is not possible."

CHAPTER 12

Lights began to flash at the edge of my eyes in February. At dinner at Ca'Dario with Vincent and Jodie, the rain pouring down in sheets, I looked outside at the street, and the puddles on the street were flashing violet. I put down the menu. I tried to behave as if everything were normal.

Flashing lights "show up," said one report on the Web. "Patients have mentioned lights that flash" after an inflammation of the optic nerve. "Photophobias," said one synopsis. "Photopsias," said another.

Vincent and I drove down to see Dr. Q, the neuro-ophthalmologist recommended by Dr. Rao. Vincent had decided he wanted to be there for every new specialist. We got an early-afternoon appointment, and Vincent figured out a route that might avoid traffic. We'd take the Five.

Dr. Q strode into the examining room with his fellow, a mild woman who practically flattened herself against the wall. He examined me. He looked at my records. He announced in a grand, all-encompassing voice, that I had had a "one-time event." It happens, he said, to people in their sixties. It would not happen again. I was greatly relieved by what he said, but I had learned, by this time, to allot a small part of myself to medical doubt. I asked him about the flashing lights.

He turned to his fellow. "Could they be . . . Charles Bonnet syndrome?" he asked her. She nodded carefully.

"Charles Bonnet," he said, "discovered that persons who had had injuries to their optic nerve sometimes suffered hallucinations; they saw 'echoes' of things that were not there anymore." He ordered an MRI.

We thanked him and walked out the door.

"It would be great if he's right," Vincent said, looking doubtful.

"Yes," I said.

On the way home, we took the Five again. It's a big freeway, four lanes each way. Near Burbank, I glanced over and saw, walking beneath the freeway wall, a hairsbreadth from the whizzing cars, a plump brown chicken, nonchalantly pecking at the ground.

I looked over at Vincent. He was driving,

hands on the wheel, staring straight ahead. I hesitated.

Just before I was about to speak, he said, "It's a chicken. On the freeway. Or maybe we both have Charles Bonnet syndrome."

I asked Dr. Burks if this could be a one-time event. She looked dubious. But we went ahead with the MRI, driving down again one Saturday morning because "the machine was better" at USC than in Santa Barbara. Dr. Q left a message on my machine after he read it that the nerve was not inflamed. He would see me in six months. When I called back to ask him questions, his office took my number, but he did not return my call. His fellow called and tried to answer my queries, but then she graduated from her fellowship.

My world remained small. I could not travel on airplanes. I had to nap at least twice a day. I could not read or work for long stretches of time. I kept my job because I needed to, but it was like holding on by the skin of my teeth. The high doses of steroids made it almost impossible to concentrate. I worked with four other people at Patagonia on the environmental team, and they made room for me — they held me up. We'd had some practice: each of them had faced a trial. Falling was not unknown to them. Still, I understood later how much they had taken on without telling me, how well they covered the extra work.

After a second visit to Dr. Rao, I was waiting for a train in Los Angeles under Union Station's beautiful carved ceiling. I had grown to love the station's tiled floors, its old leather and wood armchair seating, its garden. Out of the corner of my eye, I saw a man in a soiled overcoat peering into a garbage can. He walked in front of me, and he had a face and body that I had last seen in Nicaragua in the late 1980s, a body not of this century. The men walking along a road near Managua had been bent over double by the bundles of wood on their backs. I had taken them at first for animals. There was nothing on this man's face to cover his naked hopelessness.

My first impulse was to run after him and stuff some money in his pocket, but instead I just stood there. What was going on was something more than the usual hesitation I have before giving money to a stranger. The space between us was much smaller than it had been when I was in my former life. The world could discard me about as fast as it had (a long time ago) discarded him. I had watched people's eyes pass over me, with my swollen, red cheeks and my slightly off-balance gait. I was sick and getting old. If I lost my job, if Vincent left me . . . it would take a while in my case, and it might never come to what it had for this man, formerly a human being, but I saw the chute he had fallen down. It ran parallel, if at a distance from mine. We were both disposable.

I looked around, and with a burning hatred, I hated every single person who looked even remotely well in the whole station. I hated not only the young but the middle-aged, anyone who looked as if they were healthy. There they were, some of them talking on cell phones or just walking along, looking anxious or tense or smug. They don't know! I hated everyone who was not sick or poor. And finally I railed at God, THE FATHER ALMIGHTY. Then it came home to me, fully and completely, why the creed was so wrong. God, the Father Almighty, was the God the empire liked and wanted to adopt as its own. God the King. God the Emperor. The God I hoped was somewhere (at the zoo?) and wanted to learn to pray (to? with?) was not that God. Not your grandfather's God. I wanted another story. I needed another story.

I understood that the inflammation and

its aftermath had caused, not only a sudden descent into a separate country but a break in the narrative of my life. The narrative had been onward and upward. The narrative was that I was working to be more successful, more powerful, possibly rich. I was, after all, an American.

In my packing and talking and traveling, hidden and quiet, was my desire to be successful or, at the very least, famous. When I was given an upgrade, I liked walking on the ridiculous patch of red carpet that United Airlines puts out for its first-class passengers. I liked sauntering past the rabble. I hungered after the Chanel jackets in the *New York Times* ads. I envied the writers who sold more books than I did.

It was, if you will, the official American story: The rich got rich, and we could all get rich, too. If we weren't rich already, we were, as David Brooks once said, "Pre-rich."

Every culture produces such a story. It runs (unconscious) under daily life. It takes a crack in it to reveal its presence. I was living in the crack.

While hoping to get rich is an old American story (just ask Henry James), it has gotten out of hand. My parents did not talk about real estate and money the way we do. They talked about a fulfilled life, a meaningful job. But now wanting to get rich, coupled with a consumer culture, smothers our ability to imagine other narratives. It's like getting used to fewer and fewer trees, more and more foul air. Jared Diamond calls this "landscape amnesia."

It was summed up by a sign in Zuccotti Park during Occupy Wall Street: WORK CONSUME BE SILENT DIE.

And then, along came October 2008, when what was revealed to us in stunning detail was what the theologian Walter Brueggemann once called "the abnormality that has become business as usual." What was revealed was how banks and financial institutions, as Nicholas Kristof wrote in *The New York Times,* "socialized risk and privatized profits." The underpinning of the official story was revealed in its callousness, corruption, and criminality.

The world that Jesus inhabited had its own version of this story: King Herod, the puppet of the Romans, taxed the poor into submission; the temple authorities collaborated with the empire. There was a hierarchy, a red carpet, special clubs. The rich got rich and the poor got poorer. And the suffering was ignored, papered over, invisible. Or the poor were blamed for their poverty; the ill were blamed for being ill.

When Jesus said, "The poor will always be with you," did he not mean, *The rich will always be with you, and, thus, the poor?* When he healed a blind beggar or fed thousands on a hillside or told a young lawyer a story about carrying a wounded Samaritan to an inn, he was revealing the suffering that was business as usual. He was writing it on the walls.

Later, when I could fly again but was relegated to steerage, I stood with the rabble while first class boarded on that little piece of red polyester. I knew I would not be walking on it anytime soon. It is so trivial, but what I realized was how incredibly insulting the carpet is. That it symbolized what a stupid place we have come to. I could not see Jesus walking (or kneeling) on that red carpet. As I stood there, I saw that there was a further piece to the get-rich story. As you climbed the ladder, you would leave the people who had been standing beside you. That was the underpinning of the story: you would get rich (or famous or whatever) and walk away on the carpet and leave your old companions — the ones who had held you up — behind.

As I came down from a short, easy hike, my left leg felt weaker than the right one, and a seizing electrical pain jolted its way through the right side of my head. Dr. Mesipam sent me to a neurologist, who ordered a lumbar puncture. MS came back on the radar.

I found myself in a white room with a wide white bed, one doctor and one nurse. I was in the usual nightie, the dispiriting uniform of Oz. I was cold.

(I know that many patients are tougher than I am, but sometimes I think people describe their experiences in Oz with stoicism in order to avoid that most onerous of accusations: self-pity. We are supposed to suffer the worst tests and "procedures" with resolve and bravery, or we will be someone who has self-pity. I am not sure this is a good idea. It makes us all have to be braver and more stoical than we may feel; it diminishes our need for support; and finally, it makes the medical world think the tests and procedures aren't so bad, which is the worst result. And it's part of the battle imagery so prevalent in Oz — witness those cancer ads for Sloan-Kettering.

(Be a wimp, I say to my fellow patients. Or cultivate something other than stubborn endurance. Cultivate compassion for yourself and for others. This is a hard world, Oz, and any way you get through is a triumph.)

The doctor pulled a machine, a version of

a CT scan, until it hovered over my back. He was going to pierce my spinal cord with a needle and draw out fluid. He would find the spine with the machine, scrub some Xylocaine on the spot, and then punch through to it with a needle. I would feel "pressure."

I did. He sat back. He was pulling out the fluid. We waited. It was slow, too slow, he finally said. He told me they were going to tilt the bed. I felt it lift and tilt downward, to force the fluid out faster.

Finally he said, in the tone one might have for a frustrating household project, "I am going to have to do it again."

"Again!" I said.

"Yep," he said. "I have to find a better place."

This time it was more than pressure.

Finally he got enough fluid to send to the Mayo Clinic to be tested for oligoclonal bands, the gold standard for MS.

Vincent picked me up. I had to remain horizontal for four hours; otherwise spinal fluid could leak into the brain, and I would have a "massive" headache. Vincent would not allow me to stand up except to go to the bathroom. He served me roasted potatoes and salmon in bed and, to talk to me, knelt down on the floor and turned his head sideways.

175

I met with the neurologist. The test had come back negative for the oligoclonal bands, he told me; I could lay the fear of MS to rest. I thanked him. My symptoms were, or seemed, I said, neurological. The neurologist said I should stop worrying. It must be something farther down the nerve, he said, where we can't see. And what would that mean? I asked him. Without responding to my question, he said, "Retrobulbar neuritis. Pretty direct meaning: behind the bulb, behind the eye.

"Some kind of inflammation," he said, with a dismissive wave. "Behind the eye."

A medical paper I read about retrobulbar optic neuritis said: "The doctor sees nothing and the patient sees nothing." The doctor doesn't see the inflammation, and the patient is not aware of it, and yet it goes on.

At that point I was too inexperienced. I could have asked: "What kind of inflammation? What do people do? What category does it fall under? Or when is that not MS?" Instead I said, "Oh."

I asked Dr. Mesipam what retrobulbar neuritis meant and he replied with a wry smile, "It's inflammation, farther down the nerve, where he can't see it."

I thought at first that I should learn the

medical words tossed at me: *retrobulbar neuritis, edema.* But I found that when I used them, many doctors frowned and pulled back.

Better to say "swollen." Better not to refer to something found on the Internet.

The neurologist wanted to taper the prednisone again. Dr. Burks agreed, but she was worried about moving too fast. After all, she said, a refrain, we still don't really know what we're dealing with.

My former life had been fueled by adrenaline and anxiety, in equal amounts. I ran just ahead of what was overcoming me. When I took a day or two off, I was restless and bored, and the world was pale and flat. Glued to my screen, I lived in two dimensions. But now I was slower, and parts of the world, its creatures, its particles, started to enter my diary: *yellow-breasted birds in the plum tree. It's quiet, as if summer were just around the corner.*

As I had nowhere else to travel, I watched the creek restoration's progress. One day it was complete. The road was open, the equipment gone. A plastic green fence was stitched along the periphery of the area, to protect new native grasses and plants. I found a place where the fence ended and walked over to the creek.

I threaded my way past new hummingbird sage and penstemon. I could see the pool before I got to it. In the clear winter light that marks February in California, when everything stands out as if it were posing for an Ansel Adams photograph, the pool was deep and green. Clean, brown sand lay along its edge. A sycamore tree, empty of leaves, stood across from me, its white-gray bark glimmering. Along the edge, and jutting into the creek, the restorers had placed large, flat rocks. I looked up and down the creek, and I could see a series of pools, a series of rocks. Should the steelhead ever return from the place of near extinction, they would have deep clear pools in which to spawn. I sat down.

For the first time in a very long time, I felt my shoulders relax.

CHAPTER 13

It was now mid-February. Vincent and I were united in our desire to discover what had caused the nerve inflammation, and how best to treat it.

I sensed that many of the people around us, apart from those closest to us, wanted us to "move on."

"I'll bet this is just about the nerve and nothing systemic," a friend said. I wondered if he did not know how to deal with something so . . . what was the word? Ongoing. Neither did I.

Illness, like other parts of the official story, was something you got over. It was a challenge you overcame. You were big, it was small. I knew this was not the case. It was big, you were small. The medical world was full of mystery and confusion. Doctors were often baffled; the system of specialists who did not follow up on patients made it worse.

I imagined the lives of doctors, these

people who worked in Oz but were not sick. How did they manage? How did they defend themselves against the fear and vulnerability and illness that surrounded them, the sure knowledge that it would happen to them (they know the body, after all), the slow, inevitable slide toward death? (I had a moment in a doctor's office of imagining that she saw me from the inside out, like the pictures on examining room walls: the lower intestine, the pancreas, the gall bladder.)

When a doctor did not know what was wrong or felt on tenuous ground, I discovered, he or she often became irritated with the patient. It was your fault that you had a mysterious disease.

When I told a resident at Doheny that the bright blobs of color were increasing, he replied, "Your vision is the best we will see today." (A coincidence, Vincent said later. "Yours was the worst bedside manner we saw all day.")

The more experienced and confident the doctor, the less defensive he or she was. The doctors who managed to be the least defensive were the men and women who worked in autoimmune disease.

An expert in rheumatology at UCLA ordered more blood tests from her own lab, which, it turned out, was a better lab than my local one. (A surprise: some labs are better than others.) She ordered, without telling me, a test for neuromyelitis optica, or Devic's disease, an autoimmune disorder that attacks the eyes and spinal column. Devic's can blind a person, lead to seizures and paralysis. Dr. Hahn knew there was a new, definitive blood test for it. Only when it came back negative did she tell me of her concern.

Dr. Hahn asked what I did for work and inquired about my novel. I told her it took place in New Mexico when they were building the atom bomb. I would send the book to her, I said, feeling sure I would not hear of it again. The next time I saw her, she told me she had read it with pleasure and that Arthur Compton, the physicist, had been her patient in St. Louis toward the end of his life.

She told me that she did not know exactly what I had but wondered about a rare lung autoimmune disease. She would ask for a consultation with a pulmonary specialist at UCLA. He never replied.

I still had the seizing electrical pulses on the right side of my head, especially after exercise, and bursts of electricity, like a burst of a burn, in my legs and in my hands. I had pain at the back of my head and in my temples. My visual field deteriorated when we tapered the prednisone. The weird blobs of color continued at the periphery of my right eye and sometimes, frighteningly, at the edge of my left, "good" eye. I would be walking to the park, and what seemed like the northern lights would go off at the edge of the eye. New sharp lights began to appear closer to the center of my vision, bright red stars. Dr. Rao ordered a blood test for antiretinal antibodies, and I tested positive for two. Now I was in a zone where almost no doctor had experience.

"What are these new antibodies?" I asked Dr. Hahn as she faced me, feeling along my throat.

"Another thing, maybe."

"Is it one of those things in the gray zone?"

She looked up and into my eyes. "Very gray."

It was now spring. I made an appointment with Dr. Mesipam and sat in his waiting room in a soft, overstuffed chair. A man near me was watching the stock market on his iPad. His wife, wearing a tawny cashmere sweater and soft sweatpants, had a bruise on her face from falling, she told Sarah, the receptionist, after being released from the hospital.

I told Dr. Mesipam that I had been thinking about how so many people were sicker than I was. Maybe I should give up searching for a diagnosis. "After all —" I started.

He interrupted: "Just because you are walking around doesn't mean you aren't sick," he said. "This is about your sight. It's about your eyes."

Meanwhile daily life went on as much as it could. In my notebooks were questions regarding our small nest egg, lists of what kind of headsets to buy to work with Skype, followed by "lesions on nerve, scars." Then, "Blue Star stoves."

Merrill Lynch
Toilet Paper
Laundry Soap
Blood Test

Other, larger questions loomed. "If we don't go to Maine" was written in one notebook. "What about Claire's wedding?"

The right words and the wrong words continued to preoccupy me as never before, even after thirty years of writing. The right word pierced the wall between my world and the other one. The wrong one hardened and reinforced it. The larger world that I was no longer a character in contained many wrong words. There were of course the words of ads and commercials, which seemed to be taking place not only in another country but on another planet, but also the words people said in passing: "Hang in there." "How are you?"

Along with people who sent the wrong words in my direction were the people who used the right ones. My friend Harriet referred in an e-mail to my "living nightmare."

"I've been thinking of you," said my friend Elizabeth, whose sister had been ill for years. "As I walked in the park yesterday, I thought of how we are all so fragile, so vulnerable." What she said not only contained the word *we* but also was a recognition of our tragic actual reality. The thing I was experiencing that most people wanted not to see.

Not to see that reality, I understood, was not to see me.

I once interviewed Jews who had recently emigrated from Russia in one of the openings in the Cold War in the 1980s. Many of them had survived the siege of Leningrad. They were living in a retirement home in Denver. One of them took me aside after I had been there for a few days and said, "Tell me, Nora. Is everyone in America always fine? I ask someone how they are doing and they reply, always, 'Fine.' "

I explained to her that this was a commonplace; a custom, it meant nothing. Relief showed all over her face.

"Ah," she said. "That's good. Because I am rarely fine." (Later, whenever they saw me, they would chorus: "How are you? We are fine!" and then laugh uproariously.)

I missed them, I thought. These were people who understood not fine.

After several months of not going to church, I felt aimless. And I missed communion.

I decided to return to the base community, a small group of people who tried to follow a pattern of reading the Bible like the base communities formed in Latin America in the 1960s. After the Latin American bishops conference at Medellín, Colombia, in 1968, base communities became part of liberation theology: the theory was that God has a "preferential option" for the poor and the outcast over the wealthy and powerful. Liberation theology, in turn, was influenced by Paulo Freire, a Brazilian, author of *Pedagogy of the Oppressed.* Freire created a way for peasants to learn how to read and also to recognize

185

the constraints placed on them.

A story goes that one of his students, a peasant woman in Rio Grande do Norte, read aloud a newspaper article about the exploitation of salt in her area. A visitor asked her, "Do you know what *exploitation* means?"

She replied, "Perhaps you, a rich young man, don't know. But I, a poor woman, I know what exploitation is."

The base community at Trinity met on Thursdays at noon, read the gospel story for the next Sunday, then talked about its meaning in their lives. They asked how it was speaking to each one of them. What did it ask them to do? Sometimes they asked themselves which person in the story of the gospel was the person with whom they most identified. They were hardly powerless peasants trying to understand the workings of God in their daily lives, or how this might relate to a larger justice, but I had been in a base community before, and I knew it was a place to talk seriously with a group of people about how to live. What followed the conversation was a brief communion, using the "reserved sacrament," wafers and wine that had already been blessed by a priest. We passed them around to each other.

The base community was mainly a

middle-class crew: a retired professor of social work; a professor of classics; my old friend Ann Jaqua, a spiritual director; a real estate appraiser; a friend who grew up in the South, a Methodist; another who grew up in an evangelical church but was gay and had to leave.

The New Testament reading the first week I returned was about a man who was ill and lying beside the temple pool. An angel of God descended unannounced into the pool and "roiled the waters." If you jumped in while the waters were roiling, you were healed.

The problem for this man was that he could not walk or, presumably, roll, so someone else was always getting there before him.

He had been there for thirty-three years.

As we went around the table, the other people were, to my amazement, critical of the man.

"Why didn't he get some help?" one asked.

"Thirty-three years," said another. "You'd think he'd figure it out by then."

"When I have a sore ankle," said another, "I walk on it and it feels better."

When my turn came around, I said that I understood why he had not been able to get help during the thirty-three years — he had been dealing with specialists.

No one laughed. The expressions on their faces ranged from concern to perplexity. I understood that I was very angry. I was angry at them and angry at the doctors and angry angry angry.

But I continued to go to the community. I talked, hesitantly, and then with more confidence, about the feeling of being isolated. Those people in the gospel stories — the blind beggar, the deaf-mute, the paralytic — they were not only sick, I understood, they were alone.

In that room, my story did not always fit into the larger one, but my *derrotero* had a coastline similar to parts of the larger map. I was not unlike the man desperate to get into the roiling water; I was afraid of becoming the blind beggar. The stories pitched into the places in me I was afraid to reveal. The others had stories, too. Each week we grappled with the gospel readings, and some truths rose up. One week the reading was Matthew 10:40–42: "Anyone who welcomes you welcomes me, and anyone who welcomes me welcomes the one who sent me. . . . And if anyone gives even a cup of cold water to one of these little ones who is my disciple, truly I tell you, that person will certainly not lose their reward." Ann Jaqua said, "Something about the water makes me think of how connecting to the person in need of water connects us to Jesus and then to God. God comes to us, not only in Jesus but in simple acts of compassion to the 'others.' It has an oceanic feeling about it."

When I saw Mark Asman one day outside the library on my way out the door, I told him I felt guilty that I wasn't going to church. He replied, "Not going to church? What do you call the base community? I think it might be proper to say, you're not going to Sunday church."

I still found the right words in the books I listened to. I finished *The Death of Ivan Ilyich* and *Anna Karenina*. And read *Great Expectations*. The great nineteenth-century writers continued to show me, as *New York Times* columnist Judith Warner said, "that little bit of raggedness that for some of us is really the heart of what makes us human." My life, in its raggedness, was part of a large, ongoing, messy creation. I was not alone in my fear and failure to "conquer" my situation, my rage, and my helplessness. And yet as much as the novel *Anna Karenina* had raggedness, it also had a moral center. Not an Aesop's fable with a proverb at the end, but a coherence, an order, that despite its tragic end made me feel more alive. If I believed in anything, I believed in the life of the imagination.

My friend Gary Hall, the dean in Washington, had headed a seminary before moving to his current post. The seminary was failing, and it turned out that Gary's job was to close it down. As he worked through the final days of the school, with grieving staff and students, he said that he turned, not to the prayer book or to the Bible, but to Shakespeare's plays. The two that meant the most to him were *The Winter's Tale* and *The Tempest.*

The Winter's Tale was important for two reasons: it represents real, pointless human malignity, and it also enacts a kind of resurrection scene when the statue of Hermione comes to life. *The Tempest* was important for a similar and a new reason. There is all this human enmity in the play, and the process the play ritualizes leads to a deep acceptance/forgiveness that our liturgy only performs in a thin, pro forma way. The other thing, new to me, was the transformation Prospero goes through. The standard rap on Prospero is that he is like Shakespeare, manipulating all the characters in a meta-theatrical event.

What struck me really deeply in 2008 was the way in which Prospero himself is healed by the ritual. He is able, at the end, to throw off his power and forgive those who have betrayed and wounded him. I found both plays extremely powerful, much more so than chapel. So did the students.

I think part of the power of the plays is the way they represent both the depths of human sin and the power of a new community "based on trust instead of threats," as W. H. Auden says of *Measure for Measure.* Part of what I had to do at the seminary was find a way to give up being enraged at my predecessors for digging us into this mess. . . . At the end, you have to assent to life and to what is. The Shakespeare plays helped me (and the entire community) do that in a way the liturgy really couldn't.

I did not know what "God" I believed in at this point. But I understood Jodie when she said one day, "I believe in writing. I believe in words."

Dr. Burks told me that she wanted me to go on a new drug, a "steroid-sparing drug," that would ease the tapering of the pred-

nisone, she hoped. It was called methotrexate. It was "a kind of chemotherapy," having been used against breast cancer at first
and now against rheumatoid arthritis. It
would tamp down the body's ability to make
new cells. I would have to have a blood test
every month, to check my "liver function."
And, she said cautiously, "it will thin your
hair."

"Do you mean," I said, "that I will have
not only fat cheeks but also thin hair?"

She nodded. She said she was sorry. I
thought of the women I had known whose
hair had fallen out. I didn't pay enough attention to them, I thought; I did not know.

The methotrexate not only thinned my
hair, it changed its texture to something like
dry acrylic. It would have made a good
prayer shawl. But I started actually being
able to taper the prednisone below 30 milligrams. And I, who have always been afraid
of needles, got used to delivering my arm
up to the nurses in the hospital's lab every
month.

In July we finally concluded that I could
not travel to Claire's wedding in Wyoming.
We called her, and we all cried. I felt like —
I was — a sick person, one of those who
"just can't make it." I had not had enough
sympathy for them, those citizens of Oz.

We decided on a staycation, having never done one. The first week we visited local places we had always meant to see: the sand dunes north of Santa Barbara in Guadalupe (where *The Ten Commandments* was filmed); a wild beach where we walked against the wind. The second week we hired a friend's housekeeper, and the three of us cleaned together — the ash from wildfires the previous fall was in every crevice of every corner. We lingered at Sears and finally bought a new refrigerator, a thing of beauty that was far beyond the word "appliance." I got up in the middle of the night just to look at it.

When we were finished, the house felt full of light. It was inhabited.

I checked in again with Dr. Mesipam. I sat in his smallest examining room and asked him what I should do.

He replied, "Why not go to Mayo?" The legendary clinic in Minnesota.

"I have been thinking the same thing," I said. "How do I get in?"

"My batting average is about fifty-fifty," he said. "I mean, about half of the patients I have recommended get in. I have no idea what their criteria are." He and Dr. Burks both offered to write a letter.

I assembled my records. I constructed a narrative. I waited. In three weeks I got a call on my cell phone from a number that registered 507, the area code for Rochester. His name was John, at Mayo. I was to FedEx my records.

CHAPTER 14

We flew into Minneapolis. It was the first time I'd flown in ten months. Dr. Mesipam said, "After all, Mayo is there to catch you at the other end." I didn't think about the nerve as I boarded the plane. I thought about the flight's short duration and the Mayo Clinic at the other end. The people there who would catch me if I fell from space.

Rochester, Minnesota, lies about eighty miles south of Minneapolis. The day after we arrived, we drove the scenic route, down the Mississippi River, through Red Wing, home of the boots and shoes, where we stopped briefly and ate bratwurst from a street fair while sitting on a park bench a few feet from the river. Across from us were a tavern, houseboats, and a dock. Near us was a monument to those who lost their lives in a steamboat accident in 1890. Families on a summer cruise of the river, a barge towed behind the festive boat for the added people, a sudden wind. Whole families drowned. I read the monument about the accident with great concentration. I was paying attention to chance, how things come to us out of nowhere.

All Minnesota seemed to be outside in the unusually warm weather. Limestone cliffs rose up as we traveled farther south. The hillsides were red and gold. At Frontenac Park people sat at picnic tables overlooking the river; they were waiting for eagles and migrating tundra swans. We turned inland.

Outside Rochester was a sign that advertised it as the Best Place to Live in America.

As we drove into the town, past the small malls, the big malls, the fast-food joints, and then a neighborhood of two-story midwestern houses with wide porches, we could see two gray and glass high-rise buildings at the center of town. As we grew closer, signs with the immediately recognizable three-shield blue logo appeared and then the words MAYO CLINIC.

Thirty-five thousand people are employed by Mayo in a city of just over 100,000. The clinic itself is in these two twenty-story buildings, Gonda and Mayo. A thousand people a day pass through the doors.

The Kahler Inn and Suites was across the

street and down the block from Gonda. It was dowdy and privately owned and had a large TV in the small lobby, around which people who did not look well sat on a large lumpy couch watching CNN. We checked into a spacious plain room and went outside to find something to eat.

Hardly anyone seems to actually live in downtown Rochester — the Mayo buildings and hotels and restaurants that serve the sick constitute almost all of it. The downscale Kahler Inn and Suites, the upscale Marriott and DoubleTree. (The Marriott had town cars with drivers waiting outside, groups of women in head scarves and men in dark expensive suits.) The streets at night seem to be populated only by patients and their families. That first evening, we were almost run over by two elderly women driving motorized sit-down scooters. Each of them had a guard that propped her chin up, as if part of her chin or neck were missing or needed support. They were driving along the sidewalk at speed and talking about whether they were going to make the light. Each of them in her right hand held a lit cigarette.

On another block was a younger woman, chubby and dressed in a shapeless cotton dress. She too was sitting on one of the scooters, but she had a small calico cat in her lap. She smiled warmly. We smiled back. Later we would see a small group of people standing around her stroking the cat while she talked to them. The cat, I saw, was a lure.

We learned fast that almost everyone in the hotels was going to the clinic. There was really no other reason to be there. At every restaurant, at every hotel breakfast, at the smallest transaction (buying underwear, cough drops), the clerk or waitress would say to me, "Good luck," and we both knew what that meant. Soon Vincent and I said it, too, when we got off an elevator, to the people still inside.

Our dinner that first night was at a café recommended by a friend of a friend, a woman who had a stage-three cancer and is alive, she said, because of Mayo. Being alive "because of Mayo" is a refrain. Another is "It took them twenty-four hours to diagnose it." And although I don't watch *House* or the other medical TV shows (I am too scared to), the shows must have added to the expectation, the answer that all of us who are patients here, seek.

Before I fell asleep, what came to my mind was that Rochester was a cross between Lourdes and *The Magic Mountain.* I had heard of so many patients who had traveled miles and miles and waited for months to get here on a pilgrimage to healing. And having seen the women downtown that night, I wondered if, like Hans Castorp and other patients in *Magic Mountain,* there were people who were at home here or were, by a combination of illness and medical institutionalization, trapped. The whole town was Oz.

In the morning, we had our first two appointments, and the only appointments so far on my list. I was to start at the place where the symptoms started, in ophthalmology, and they would set up the next appointments within the clinic. I had heard of the famous Mayo team system but didn't really know much more than lore.

I was anxious. I dressed carefully, trying to look like a real person, a professional, a person who was more than her illness, all of which disappeared as I walked into the building.

We entered through a tunnel from our hotel, one of the many makeshift subways that connect the buildings in downtown Rochester. (The reason for them would become unmistakably apparent when we returned the following March.) We followed a young couple pushing what looked like a lump of blankets in a wheelchair. One handled the chair and the other rolled an oxygen tank alongside. As we grew closer to the glass automatic doors that opened into the Gonda Building, more and more people were walking with us: the halt and the lame and the very sick. A man on crutches. A little girl with a bald head. A man with his whole leg covered in a bandage.

In the two-story entryway were huge "chandeliers," or glass sculptures, made by Dale Chihuly — bursts of yellow and green that extended the length of the long bright hall. The glassmaker wanted them to be cheerful, he said, and I was glad that he had been commissioned to make these blasts of warm color for this place. Compare them to the usual lights found in most hospitals and lobbies of medical clinics — the cottage cheese ceilings, the cold, weird lighting fixtures that seem to have been manufactured for medical offices alone. These were made by an identifiable human hand.

From the beginning, Mayo distinguished itself in this way: it struggled against the impersonal that is the ubiquitous nature of most medical institutions. The people who built and planned the Mayo Clinic and who, I imagined, kept working at it, were trying to combine both efficiency and humanity in every Mayo transaction. They did not always succeed at this almost insurmountable task, but not for lack of trying.

Once we passed out from under Chihuly's glass, we were in a larger area. In front of us was a vast room with a glass-walled atrium planted in fall colors, red and orange. In front of the atrium was a grand piano with a small polite sign that invited anyone to play as long as you thought "people would enjoy it." No one was sitting at the piano as we walked in, but someone would play later in the week and leave me with one of my most lasting impressions of the Mayo Clinic. This lobby is two stories high. I imagined that the person who designed it hoped to counteract the feeling of being crowded.

When we walked out of the elevator onto the seventh floor, we faced a glass case containing tribal clothes from New Zealand. In every nook and corner in the Mayo Clinic buildings was original art or collections of beautiful objects: Chinese porcelain in neurology, Steuben glass in X ray, an Asian rug with a pattern of beautiful running horses in CT scan. No pastel machine-made watercolor prints.

The chairs in the ophthalmology waiting

area were comfortable and broken up by a glassed-in optometry shop. Other waiting areas were next to large glass windows with easy chairs and couches in a living room arrangement. Part of the problem with medicine is its pervasive impersonality, the way one feels as if one's singularity were slowly being eroded by the attitudes of the assistants, the doctors, and the surroundings. These attitudes were often based on the glass wall: they were on one side, we were on the other. But at Mayo, when I was there, the smallest transaction had a quality of both gentleness and competence, a vast, interlocking machine of efficiency communicated on human terms. To help the bad business of waiting, receptionists told me exactly where the doctors were. (*He is in the lab. She is with residents.*) They invited me to come to the desk "after thirty minutes of waiting." I was never given a rude or vague reply. Patients were encouraged to ask for an earlier or different appointment if time was freed up. When I arrived at one doctor's desk earlier than planned and told the receptionist, she said, "I will text him to tell him you are here. He is in the lab. When he replies, I'll let you know right away."

Lines were avoided by the large number of people behind the desks and little buzzers like those that restaurants give you to announce your table is ready. To pass the time, jigsaw puzzles were left out on square tables (my favorite touch). Free Internet and, in some areas, free computers. Televisions were small and unobtrusive.

Light was maximized. Glass walls, floor-to-ceiling windows, skylights, the entry atrium.

The staff reached toward us rather than turning away. They deemphasized the wall between us by concentrating on what we had in common. More than anything, they, with few exceptions, did not lord it over the patients; someone had thought about the power that medical staff have, innately, over the vulnerable and the sick and had done dozens of small things to counteract it.

Yet despite everything Mayo did, from the well-educated and friendly Minnesotans it employed to the jigsaw puzzles it provided, they were still "the staff" or "the doctors." They were still inhabitants of well land. We were in Oz. I longed for a doctor who had had something go wrong with her eyes.

As I sat in the waiting area, I thought about how, in my past life, I had just kept going forward, adding things to my to-do list, flying back and forth across the continent, speaking to church groups, writing, teaching, preaching, holding down a part-time job, cooking, cleaning . . . I thought about the people I knew who did this kind of thing well into their sixties, well into their seventies. Not many, but a few. Did I have an inner thermostat that ceased working, that could not adjust? Would it be "all downhill from here"? What if I did not "get well"?

My first appointments were with Dr. Leavitt, a neuro-ophthalmologist, and Dr. Herman, a specialist in uveitis. My vision was tested, my eyes were dilated. The fact that the afflicted eye did not contract properly when a flashlight was shone into it was duly noted. Not noted was the look of alarm on the technician's face, and her repeated motions with the flashlight, her calling in another technician to confirm it. Then we were shown into a comfortable examining room paneled in blond wood rather than painted white, with an examining chair next to a wide desk built into the wall. Dr. Leavitt, a small, upright woman dressed in a gray silk suit, walked in, introduced herself, and examined my eyes.

Dr. Leavitt said the nerve looked "quiet." It looked "white," as optic nerves look when they have been "assaulted." I should have another brain MRI.

In the early afternoon we saw Dr. Leavitt's colleague, Dr. Herman, a specialist in uveitis and glaucoma, with a mild midwestern face. He wore a tweed jacket and large scuffed shoes. His office too was faced in warm blond wood. Cabinets lined the walls. Mayo was working against the impersonal, right down to the jigsaw puzzles. Right down to Dr. Herman's scuffed shoes.

He asked if he might look at my eyes. He told me they were "very quiet."

"Someone said I had blepharitis," I said to him.

"Not now," he said from behind the scope.

"What are these pockets at the corners of my eyes?" I asked.

"Not to put too fine a word on it," he said, "they are fat. As the tissue thins, fat deposits."

"Could I have low-intensive glaucoma?" I asked, hesitant. I asked because one of Dr. Burks's patients who had similar symptoms to mine had discovered after six months and the wrong ophthalmologist that she had low-intensive glaucoma and was going blind.

"No," he said. "The nerve would look different. Cupped." He made a cupping motion with his hands.

He sat back in his chair. He said quietly,

"You may not find the cause of this."

I wanted to scream at him, *That is why I came here.* I believed that if I just tried hard enough, I would find the answer, especially here, at the Mayo Clinic. I would *know.*

But instead I said, "Of course." And was reminded of what Raymond Carver said automatically as he was leaving the office of the doctor who had told him he had stage-four lung cancer: "Thank you."

Toward the end of the appointment, Vincent said — it was so quiet I might have missed it — "Why can't we do the MRI today?"

When I heard him say *we,* I felt that I had been holding a heavy and unwieldy package for a year and, with one word, he took it.

Dr. Leavitt was my team captain. She had the authority to order tests and set me up with other doctors. They handed me a sheet the next morning. I was to see a rheumatoid specialist, a neurologist on two separate days, and then Dr. Leavitt again. I was to have the brain MRI and a blood test and a "twenty-four-hour urine test."

I was given a new Mayo number to replace the temporary number I had been given earlier, and it was bar-coded onto appointment sheets.

The lab area was in a "subway" floor, below the lobby. When I came out of the elevator, sheets in hand, I hesitated for a second — right or left? A man in a blue coat with a little Mayo pin appeared at my left hand and asked politely and without condescension, did I need or want direction? "Blood lab?" I said. "Right down that hall." He pointed to my right. "Straightaway." When I got there, I found ten receptionists and two people in line. Within five minutes I was in a pleasant room with a young woman who told me she would take my blood and arrange for the urine test. She asked me, as every single person who assisted me had asked, my birth date. Behind me was a miniature conveyor belt. The blood draw was painless; she placed my blood on the conveyor belt, where it rattled out of sight. Then she handed me a jug — labeled with my name and Mayo number — and told me that for the next twenty-four hours I was to pour all my urine into it. To test for heavy metals, she said. "All of it?" I said, alarmed. "All of it," she said, and smiled. "I'll give you a plastic bag to hold the urine jug," she said. I thought of the plan Vincent and I had to hike that afternoon. This will be interesting, I thought. She asked me when was the last time I ate fish of any kind (walleye, the night before), and she asked for the exact size. "Please don't eat any fish for the next twenty-four hours," she said. She looked at the clock and wrote down nine-fifteen a.m. "Tomorrow," she said, "you'll finish at nine-fifteen a.m."

"Precisely," I said.

"Precisely," she laughed.

As I left the clinic that day, I saw other people with the same plastic bag, and we silently saluted each other — united in twenty-four-hour urine. I carried the plastic bag and the jug with me into restaurants and bathrooms. In the middle of the night, I poured carefully. I balanced the bag with its jug inside in the backseat of the car on the floor. The next day, as I walked back toward a large wooden box, like an oversize crate, with URINE DROP-OFF in large letters on it, I saw a set of four interesting watercolors on the wall. I stopped to look at them, circles and squares, bright blue, orange, and yellow. They were Ellsworth Kellys.

I dropped off my urine jug, visited the Kellys again, and then saw, to my right, a frosted sliding-glass door and a sign that read CENTER FOR THE SPIRIT. The door slid open as I approached it (everything at Mayo is geared to wheelchairs). Inside was

208

a wall of wood with slots in it. A stack of blank sheets with pens and pencils on a shelf below it. Folded papers were stuck in the slots. A Wailing Wall at Mayo. Inside that room, quiet. It seemed to have been sound-proofed. I wrote a friend's name on a sheet of paper, a man who was having surgery for blocked liver ducts that day, and stuck it into one of the slots. I walked farther into the room and discovered that behind a glass partition was a small carpet printed with a labyrinth — that walking meditation path found on Cyprus and at Chartres and set in stones in Ireland.

I put my foot on the carpet and started to walk. The striking thing about labyrinths is that they are designed so the walker can't guess where in relation to the center she is. All I could do was stay where I was. The men and women who created labyrinths knew how to place the walker in the formidable present: you can do no planning in a labyrinth, you have no horizon, no way to know where you will be next.

Task: to be where I am. I was in and under the Mayo Clinic. I was buried but alive. The first thing I felt was a wash of gratitude, for all the people here at Mayo, for those who worked so hard to make it a place where the patients did not have to cope with rude receptionists, clogged medical records, and unexplained waits and could just face the things that we all were facing — what was written on the slips of paper stuck in the wall.

Then I remembered something a woman said to me when giving me a massage a few years ago, before my nerve was inflamed, when I was working at great speed. She was working on my right shoulder, and she gently said, "More going out than coming in."

I stood there on the labyrinth and thought about how I had been "spending" my life. I had been using up what savings I had as fast as I could by overworking, overextending, over, over. And now I was in debt. And the interest was pretty high, as bad as any bank's.

And I was outside the walls of the church, outside of "Christianity," in exile, in Oz. I thought about the others who had climbed over the walls of that institution, who had strayed. The ones who had said, "I can't do this anymore." We know of the big ones: Galileo, Emerson, Luther. But what about the others, the ones who one day just drifted away?

It was so much about words, I thought, as I walked on a pattern designed by persons hundreds of years ago, some of whom were members of the Catholic Church. I knew so many people by now for whom the words of the church either meant nothing or were antithetical to their experience, yet they said not a word about it. Heretics may not be tied to a stake anymore, but in any tribe our ears are tuned to the opinions of others: I voiced some doubts about the creed at a talk several years ago, and a woman stood up and walked out of the room. I thought of those for whom the words of the church were not enough, not large enough to contain their experience of the sacred. God in the rocks, in the sea, in the branches of trees. This, whispered in the hall.

As I arrived at the center of the labyrinth, a word flew straight into my mind. It was the word Vincent had said.

We.

I felt the same sensation I had felt when he said it, the shifting of a weight that I had not known I was carrying.

I pictured again the blind man in Bethsaida. He sat beside the road begging, alone. More than alone, defiled. Jesus "took him by the hand" and "led him." I had thought of this as Jesus "helping him out," or "healing" him, the holy man looking after the poor beggar. But just then I felt, rather than

211

saw, that that was not what happened that day. Instead, this blind man felt someone take his hand and walk with him. He felt someone put his hand over his eyes. He understood that someone had joined him in his suffering. Someone had said, "We."

As I left, I saw another small room with a dome-shaped skylight (where was the light coming from? we were under a twenty-story building) and realized it was meant to be a tiny mosque. Outside was a pair of shoes, and inside, a small man sat on a bench holding the Koran in one hand while checking his BlackBerry with the other.

The Kahler Inn was threadbare but homey: a laundry for guests, an odd indoor swimming pool surrounded by a wooden fence with elliptical trainers nearby, a place near the swimming pool where guests could bring food to eat at round pool-area tables. After two days at Mayo, we had a routine. Get up, have breakfast, take the subway entrance to the clinic buildings.

Every day, after the doctors' appointments or tests were completed, and after I had come back to the hotel and fallen onto the bed with appointment-going/waiting/talking-to-doctors fatigue, we went on an outing. Even though Mayo was the most sympathetic and organized of medical institutions, it was still a place where the energy required to negotiate the terrain was immense, like speaking French all day long. And where all you wanted to do was get out into "normalcy," into the oblivious world, into something else. We feared being sucked into the whole world of Mayo, generous, courteous, and nice as it was. *The Magic Mountain.* Oz. We feared never leaving.

We drove to Mayowood, the family home of the Mayos, completed in 1911, where we joined a group of midwestern women and men dressed in bland knits and one mother and daughter, in sleek athletic suits, who were probably Mayo patients. The daughter's body had a slight lack of symmetry (something was wrong), and her mother had a furrow between her eyes. It was a house with "no particular architecture," as the Mayo Clinic says. Big veranda, lots of open rooms, spacious airy bedrooms upstairs. The house was built by Charles Mayo, who founded the Mayo Clinic with his brother, William Mayo, and other doctors. The Clinic grew out of a group medical practice their father, also William, established after he returned from the Civil War. William was a small man. His wife would ask soldiers returning from the front if they had seen a doctor, and if they replied that they had seen a short one, she knew he was still alive.

We visited a bank designed by the architect Louis Sullivan in Owatonna. ("Do you have a lotta money?" Vincent asked me as we drove across the flat prairie. "No, I owe-a-tonna.")

We hiked along the Root River. We walked from our hotel to the lake in town.

Midweek we had a neurology appointment with Dr. Clarke Stevens, a gentle Canadian who walked in, washed his hands at a little sink, sat down, and then said, "Did I wash my hands?" I told him he had. He smiled. He too wore tweed.

Dr. Stevens was specific. He had read the MRI. The T-2 signals were much reduced. This meant, he said without condescension, that the nerve was better. Not completely back to "normal" but better. There was some "atrophy." It's smaller, he said, normal for a nerve that has been inflamed.

"What can we rule out?" I asked him.

"It's probably not MS," he said. "In MS usually the retinal vessels will go altogether. The white patches on the MRI were not distributed for MS." Nevertheless he would send the results to the MS team at Mayo for a consult.

"An inflamed nerve," he said, "is not usual with uveitis. It's not lupus. It's not Lymes."

It was unlikely to be ischemic (Dr. Q's "one-time event") or related to circulation.

He told me I was always welcome to call him. Which to my astonishment, several months later, turned out to be true. He told me I was always welcome to come back to Mayo.

At our last visit with her, Dr. Leavitt said that 95 percent of the optic neuritis cases they saw at Mayo were MS.

"Ninety-five percent!" I said.

"Well," she said, waving her hand in the air, "high nineties. Inflammation," she said, "opens up the blood/brain barrier."

Later I would read with some relief, "Prednisone seals it off."

They would call it "optic neuritis." Dr. Herman suggested a slow taper of 2.5 milligrams every three to four weeks down to 5 milligrams, then possibly an increase in the methotrexate. He suggested holding the taper of the prednisone at 5. "For some reason," he mused, "patients flare at five." I should have a visual field test every month.

I did not have Cogan's syndrome (different type of inflammation; hearing loss would be profound) and had no evidence of toxins, temporal arteritis, or scleritis. The check for heavy metals (twenty-four-hour urine) was negative. The pelvic X-ray that checked for spondylarthritis was negative.

It was almost a year later.

In the end, even though they had not found the actual cause, I felt that Mayo had eliminated much of what could be eliminated. I felt comforted because I had been to Mayo, and they had told me I had optic neuritis, that I was on the right drug protocol. Vincent said, "I don't think they care about the diagnosis. What they care about is things seem to be stable."

Maybe we were out of the woods, I thought. Maybe we were on the home stretch.

Just after those final appointments, we were walking quickly through the great hall, skirting people, heading for the elevators, when my eye caught a man at the grand piano. Behind him was the wall of glass that framed the outdoor atrium. In the atrium people were reading or sitting with their faces turned upward toward the rapidly diminishing sun. The man was wearing green scrubs, as if he were either about to go into an operating room or had just left one. He had a small goatee. By sitting in scrubs at the piano, he had one foot in the medical world and the other, somehow, with us in Oz.

He had just started playing the Moonlight Sonata. I stopped. He played beautifully. His concentration was complete. The music filled the space. I saw that Vincent had caught the pianist's eye and was nodding to him, a gratitude nod, and the man nodded solemnly back. Most of the people walking through the lobby just kept on going. We stood still. Then, in the atrium behind the pianist, I saw a small boy. He had the narrow shoulders and skinny legs that mark little boys, and he was running with his arms opened wide into the air. His head was bald.

The longer I resided in Oz, the more I understood how fragile life is. But in that moment, with the sonata floating in the air, the man in his scrubs working to play it well, and the boy, a piece of straw in the wind, I felt it altogether, completely.

Vincent turned, and we looked at each other, and what was transmitted between us was the shock and fear and grief and gratitude that had collected so far that year that could not be, or as yet had not been, put into words.

CHAPTER 15

After we had been home from Mayo about a month, in late November, it was time for a follow-up CT scan for the spot in my lung. I did it without thinking. There had been so many negatives on tests, this would be just another. I was therefore unprepared for the phone call from Dr. Wright, who told me that the spot in my lung had "increased in size." From 1.2 to 2 centimeters. I remembered the phrase in the medical literature regarding lung cancer: "larger than two centimeters." Dr. Wright recommended a needle biopsy.

I asked Dr. Mesipam. "It's not cancer," he said, "but I don't think a biopsy is a bad idea. We'll find out what it is."

Jodie put her life aside for that morning and took me to Pueblo Radiology. The doctor who sat us down to talk looked like a surfer, with wavy brown hair and firm shoulders. Jodie and I decided he was easy on the eyes. I got into the ubiquitous calico gown and lay down on the table in a sterile room. The entry point was in my upper left back. He would find the lesion or whatever it was with the use of a CT scan. He would numb the area going in, but there was a rib, he warned me, very near. He would use a smaller needle first and then a larger one, the one with the bore that would remove tissue. He began. He might, he said again, hit the rib. He did. The pain shot through me from my upper back straight down to my ankle. I screamed. He said, "That was the rib." He used the smaller needle to inject more Xylocaine into the hole.

He spent quite a bit of time centering the CT scanner, then inserted the larger needle. It was quick.

In a recovery room the size of a closet, I thought all was well. Jodie sat on at the bottom of the little bed rubbing my feet. They X-rayed my chest — the lung was inflated. Jodie took me home.

In the morning I walked back to Pueblo Radiology to have my lung checked. It had collapsed. Air from the collapsed lung had collected in my chest. That air was now pressing on the lung, causing it to remain collapsed. A doctor named Wrench, a name I particularly found appropriate not because he wasn't careful but because of what he had to do, told me they would have to put a tube through my chest wall. Lungs cannot be sutured; one must wait for the lung to heal on its own. "We never operate on a lung to close a puncture," Dr. Wrench said. "Not even after a gunshot wound."

"Putting a tube through my chest" does not convey the tiny operating room, the fact that I was unprepared, the lack of sedative, the nurse who held my hand. The tube allowed air to leak slowly out of the chest cavity so that the lung could expand.

Once that air escaped through the tube, the lung could expand and, Dr. Wrench hoped, remain that way. He showed me a valve on the tube; it would remain open, and if the lung expanded, he would close it and then wait four hours to see if it remained inflated. If it remained full, he would take the tube out.

After he was finished, I walked out the door. "Take the elevator," one of the nurses called after me.

I walked down the street, the plastic tube hanging off my chest under my jacket. I looked like one of those women who had too much plastic surgery in the movie *Brazil*. The end of the tube wasn't covered. I kept thinking that some kind of bacteria would get in.

I walked behind several medical buildings (The Eye Center, Physical Therapy Parking), along a sidewalk where there was a new wooden bench, passed a new parking "structure," and then skirted a small broken-down garage in which someone had parked an ancient green VW. I always took this route to get to my appointments in order to see the garage and the VW, which, because they were not medical or new or impersonal, always cheered me up.

I felt more behind the glass wall than I had in many months. Farther into Oz. Over the last two days I had had a needle pushed through my back and into my lung, then an incision in my chest while I was awake, through which plastic had been pushed, leaving me with a piece of tubing resting on my chest.

When I got to our house and ran a glass of water, my hand shook. I felt deeply uncertain of who I was. With obliviousness, with the faith that my body would always be trustworthy, went part of my identity. I was alone in an empty house with a collapsed lung.

Much worse things had happened to others. I thought of the small bald boy at Mayo.

I thought of people who had been tortured. My mind knew the difference between someone deliberately inflicting pain and someone inflicting pain in order to help, but I wondered if my body knew it.

I remembered giving the novel to Dr. A and how I had thanked him for ten minutes of his time.

Giving the novel to Dr. A, I understood, had been my way of asking for recognition that I had a profession apart from that of patient. No, more than that. That I was a *person*.

Every day I walked over to Pueblo Radiology. Every day the lung had expanded, and they shut off the valve. And every day when I walked back at noon, the lung had collapsed again. The puncture wasn't healing. A week later Dr. Burks would say that she thought it was the steroids. I was on 20 milligrams of prednisone. Her mentor, she said, had taught her that if someone was on 30 milligrams of prednisone, he would never do open lung surgery because the lung would not heal.

One day after the biopsy, the surfer doctor passed through the X-ray area where I was having my daily scan. He said, almost in passing, running his hands through his thick hair, "I don't know. I certainly thought I got it." I didn't understand what he meant. I would understand later.

I opened an e-mail from Dr. Wright, and he told me that the pathology report had come back negative. I felt a wide expansion of feeling, a sudden expansion of air and light. I walked around my study with my arms folded around myself, holding my lung, my chest, my body.

"But," Dr. Wright said, "we will have to follow this."

Finally, on Monday at noon, eleven days after the biopsy, the lung remained expanded. I saw it in my mind's eye as a miracle of tissue that took in and held air.

Just before I had the tube removed, I had an appointment with Dr. Wright. He showed me the pathology report. He drew a circle on a piece of paper.

"The lesion is here. We'll follow up," he said, "with a PET scan."

"I don't think I want to do a PET scan," I said. "So much radiation."

I did not understand, then, what he was saying. I was still involved with the tube. The tube was the thing on the front burner.

"What if the lung collapses again after they remove the tube?" I asked.

"It won't," he said.

"I think I should wait until tomorrow," I said.

He looked at me carefully.

"I think you should walk over there and have it removed," he said. "Every hour it remains in there, we increase the risk of infection."

"All right," I said.

Dr. Wrench was on call. He took me back to the small room where he had put the tube in. He told me he was not going to numb the area, that I really did not need it. I looked at him skeptically. I tried not to look at the coil of tubing on my chest. He kept up a patter about the weather, a helicopter pad the hospital was building.

"What is it that you do for a living?" he asked as he approached the table.

"I am a writer," I said.

"Ah," he said as pulled on plastic gloves. "I am now going to remove all the paraphernalia that goes with this, and then I'll stop and we'll talk about how to do the final removal." He was uncoiling tubing, removing gauze.

"When I used to see a patient who had been admitted to the emergency room," he said, "I would read an account of what the patient had said and done and what the doctor thought. Now what I get are the results of tests. I used to have a story, an understanding. Sometimes I can't figure out what happened to the patient. I think medicine has lost the narrative."

He said, "Now, we're going to practice. You breathe in, and then breathe out, and when you breathe out, I'm going to remove the tube. But we're going to practice first."

"Got it," I said.

I breathed in, and then I breathed out, and he made a motion toward the tubing but did not remove it.

"Okay?" he said.

"Okay," I said.

"Now for the real deal," he said. "Breathe in."

I did.

"Now out," he said. I did, and with a motion so quick I didn't see it, he pulled the tube out. I felt exactly nothing. He covered the incision with gauze and taped it down.

"That was nothing," I said, aware suddenly that I had tears running down my cheeks, from the anxiety, from his kindness and care, from the week.

He removed his glove, put out his hand, and covered mine.

"Good for you," he said.

That night I watched a musical on TV. I felt

light and buoyant. I called Jodie to tell her the tube was out, then mentioned that I had thought about leaving it in overnight, "in case," I said, "the lung collapsed again."

She said, alarmed, "Do you think you might be imagining the worst out of defensiveness or just because —"

"I don't imagine the worst —" I began then thought better of it. I imagined the worst out of the realization that the worst, or some version of it, happens. The nerve is inflamed. The lung collapses. The doctors don't know what the "narrative" is. By that time, I knew that doctors routinely bullshitted about what lay at the other side of "surgery," "tests," "procedures," "discomfort."

It was not in my nature to imagine the worst. My nature, I now realized, was to imagine the best-case scenario and to be stoic, like my mother and her Scottish forebears. I had watched her march right through a needle biopsy of her jaw without so much as a flinch. But I had learned in this last year that imagining the best case is naïve. The best-case scenario is a way for the medical world to deal with the human suffering caused by medical intervention, so that those who cause or watch the suffering — the doctors, the nurses — can escape feelings of inadequacy and guilt. To be stoic is to suffer in silence so you can be a popular patient, which will get you nowhere.

The thin veil of invulnerability that covers most of us without knowing it had been torn. I knew that things happen. The lesion grows; the lung collapses. If I had run across the street to save the dog two seconds later . . .

Jodie and I went on to other things. I hung up. I realized I was upset. I started to cry. I called her back.

"Oh God, I am sorry," she said. She was crying, too. "But I want to say, I have to say, what are you doing to get your mind into another place besides worrying?"

I wasn't doing very much, I had to admit. Not very much at all.

At night I made lists of what to say to the doctors and what they had said to me. I heard again what they had said. "The nerve is very white." "I have never seen a nerve so white in which the patient wasn't blind."

After Jodie and I hung up, I thought again, *What is prayer? What is it for?* The various "prayers" I kept up in the middle of the night did not vanquish the constant worry. How could I find a place that was not "imagining the worst"? Or a place that was different from this, as my friend had said, "living nightmare"?

Three days later, thanks to Jodie's concern, I dragged myself to the altar area at Trinity at seven in the morning and sat down in the dark with four other people and a candle. Mark Benson at Trinity had started this "sit," this "centering prayer." It was basically a meditation, in silence, begun and ended when Mark rolled a wooden paddle along the edge of a brass bowl and it rang out into the silence. I sat for thirty minutes. Mark Asman was sitting a few chairs down. An Episcopal monk I knew was across from me. A woman who had lupus. Her husband. I just about went out of my mind. I worried, I fretted. I thought about my bills, my to-do list, the cat box uncleaned at home. My symptoms, the doctor's appointments, my mounting bills. Then I went over all of it again. Then Mark rubbed the side of the bowl for a second time, and the sound came out in waves, like ripples in a pool of water. The session was over.

The next week I went back.

In early January 2011 I finally got the pathology report, having asked for it in December, having not received it, and having had to ask for it again. I read it. I read it again. Then I called the pathologist.

"Is this saying what I think it's saying?" I said. "That the doctor at Pueblo Radiology missed the lesion in my lung?" I remembered the surfer doctor who had done the biopsy saying, "I thought I got it."

"That about says it," the pathologist said. "Yes, that says it." A pause. "Happens often," he continued. "Small, you know. Hard to get."

I sat back in my chair. The words *all for naught* walked through my brain. Then I called Dr. Wright.

"I did not understand," I said, "what you were trying to tell me. But now I think I do. The pathologist has told me. He missed the lesion."

"Yes," Dr. Wright said.

"And that's why you want to follow up with a PET scan."

"Yes," he said.

"Okay," I said.

Right before I did the PET scan, I consulted Dr. Mesipam.

"Don't do it," he said. "Don't have a PET scan. It will back us into a corner." I listened to him, but I had already scheduled it. I did not want to unschedule. I did not want to explain why to Dr. Wright. I wanted to do what I said I would do.

Between the time of knowing that they

had missed the lesion, and the PET scan, Vincent and I went up to a valley in northern Washington to stay with my first cousin, Nan, and her husband, Craig, in their cabin in the snow. We flew on an airplane. I carried a suitcase. I did what I used to do without too much thought: I joined my beloved family in the mountains. I had not seen them since the whole thing began. When I saw Nan standing outside her door, I climbed out of the car and stood beside it, my hands reaching toward her. She stretched out her hands toward me.

We skied together on long groomed tracks. We watched the ice float on the river. I felt my lungs breathe in and breathe out.

One night Craig called me to the front porch.

"Look," he said, "Orion."

"Now," he said, "come to the back porch."

I followed him.

"Look," he said, "the Big Dipper."

I did the PET scan at seven forty-five in the morning at the same cancer center where I had once taken my mother. The same calico curtains on the windows, the same soft voice of the same receptionist. A woman sat in the room with me. We were both silent. An elderly man came in with a golden retriever. The dog wagged its way across the room. We both put our hands down. The man sat down next to the woman, introduced himself as a volunteer, and asked her why she was there. She told him she was waiting for her son to have his scan. He had, she said, testicular cancer.

Then he came over to me. He was like Mr. Dick in *David Copperfield,* someone vaguely loony, harmless, and kind, exactly the right attributes for a person to help here in the doomsday room.

I told him in the bravest voice I could find, "I am having a scan because they found a lesion in my lung."

After he left, to set up a table outside, the woman and I talked to each other — his goal, I realized had been to break our particular ice. A nurse came out to get me. The woman wished me luck.

The nurse led me back to a small room with a large lounge chair. Her manner was abrupt. She said she would return. In her hands, when she came back, was a can, somewhat larger than a soup can, but made of tungsten. Her hands were covered with heavy gloves. They would "administer" this. They hooked me up to an IV and the can. I would wait for half an hour. Then they would do the scan.

After it was done, I went home and felt

sick all over. I lay down and tried to keep my mind from worrying. The next day, as I was driving home, I saw that I had a message on my cell phone. I pulled over. It was Dr. Wright. "The PET scan is abnormal," he said. "We need to talk. Make an appointment with my office tomorrow morning. I want you to bring your husband with you."

I had a brief image of surgery, chemotherapy, a bald head, but all of it fell apart. I thought: *I am not up for this.*

The next morning, having turned our lives upside down to get there, we sat across the table from Dr. Wright. He pulled up the scan on his computer. He showed us the glowing point on the upper left lung. He said, "It's hot. Not hot hot but hot. I am obligated to tell you that the radiologist thinks it's cancer. I do not."

"Why?" I said.

"Forty years of practice," he replied.

Then he said to Vincent, "If she were my wife, I'd take it out."

■ ■ ■ ■

PART THREE:
RECALLED TO LIFE

■ ■ ■ ■

CHAPTER 16

We walked together out of Dr. Wright's office. We had told him we wanted twenty-four hours to think about it. We drove to work. A wedge biopsy would mean open lung surgery. It would mean risking an incision that did not heal. I was still on steroids. I was on methotrexate, which reduces one's ability to fight bacterial infections. A friend, without a compromised immune system, had an infection from back surgery in the same hospital go to his heart. I had an image of staying in that hospital for weeks while the chances of infection went up. Was I imagining the worst out of defensiveness?

I called Dr. Mesipam. When I walked in, I said to him, "Now I know why you didn't want me to have a PET scan." He nodded, sober.

He said, "A patient of mine, a woman your age, was found to have a lit area in her lung on a PET. They did a lobectomy, went through it thin section by section, and found nothing. Then another, an eighty-seven-year-old woman, smoked like a chimney, lost twenty pounds in two months. PET found a mass in her lung. I called her son and told him to take her home, make her comfortable, no surgery, she would never make it off the table. But she said no — she wanted to know what it was. So they stuck a needle in it and found exactly nothing. She lived another ten years, smoking all the time."

He paused. "So I don't trust PETs. They light up when they're not anything, but everyone reacts to them, of course, and it backs you into a corner.

"No one," he added, "in his right mind is going to let you walk away from this scan."

"What would you do," I asked, "if you were me?"

"I would wait," he replied. "Two months. It's still below two centimeters. Have a CT scan then."

I walked out relieved and terrified.

The next afternoon Ann Jaqua and I walked over to the place in the park where they had restored the creek. We picked our way across the new plants, trying not to step on them. I could hear the water falling into the biggest pool. We passed a man sitting in a lawn chair, reading. Tiny birds hopped about in the sycamore tree. We sat down on two large rocks, placed so they overhung the pool. This little place was a scrap of nothing. It had no large views, no magnificent settings. It was not famous. I glanced at the man reading. He seemed relaxed, at home.

Ann looked at me anxiously. The night before I had had two dreams. In one a Hispanic man was driving down the road with me, and there was a branch blocking it. He said, "We should get this out of there."

In the second, a hippie medicine man said, "I would leave it alone."

"Well," Ann said, "at least your unconscious is working on it."

Just before the PET scan, I had felt as if I were reclaiming parts of my living self and parts of the living world. Skiing in the mountains, going to meetings at work, even having dinner with friends, I sometimes forgot my fear of losing my sight. The visual field test before I left for the mountains had been stable. Perhaps we could begin tapering the prednisone again. But when Dr. Wright said, "The PET scan isn't normal," I fell back into Oz. The other world — full of forward motion, plans made by the living, with certainty that this would last forever — was gone. The wall came back, heavy and thick. And with it, a new, peculiar silence.

I got out of bed. I went to work. I walked with Ann. I made love to Vincent. In short, I went on living. This was not because I was especially brave or a "trouper," another word I had erased from my vocabulary. I went on living because living is a habit. In *War and Peace,* a young Russian facing a French firing squad reaches back to loosen his blindfold, minutes before it will not make a whit of difference whether it is tight or loose or falling off.

It was a pretense of living. Only part of me was there. The rest was in that other world that we pretend does not exist: the world inhabited by people who know not only that the body will give out but exactly how it will. I understood this was the essence of Oz.

Ann and I sat there, beside the running creek, and I slowly realized that the creek, now restored to close to its original self, felt more alive.

I once spent quite a lot of time interviewing an architect, Christopher Alexander, author of *A Pattern Language.* I watched him and his crew build a house. Alexander was a tall Englishman with a barrel chest; he wore a corset under his plain oxford shirts to keep a bad back in place. His background was in chemistry and mathematics. The first day I spent with him, he was drawing leopards on a piece of plywood for tiles he planned to make for a young couple in Albany, California, near Berkeley, where Alexander taught at the university.

"You know gargoyles?" Alexander asked me. "The heads, the beasts, and the saints that stick out from walls? I think they represent things from the Bible. In any case, they are certainly not polite. In many cases, they are placed where no one can see them. On a vault's upper side, for example, or on a piece of wall invisible to someone unless they're standing two hundred feet off the ground, or in the valley between a roof and a wall so you couldn't find them unless you're mending the roof. I think the mason who made such a gargoyle made it as part of his consecration of his stonework, and it was irrelevant whether it was seen." Alexander, an atheist, said, "I have a feeling he meant it to be seen only by God."

The leopards he was drawing would decorate a floor of a long room that looked out into a garden. They would be made of some sort of clay, Alexander thought. Each one would be shorter than the hand of a medium-size person. Because the room was 250 feet square, the leopards might be lost in it, but Alexander didn't think so. Like the gargoyles in the eaves, he thought the leopards might not be seen, but they would be felt.

On the walls of his own living room in the Berkeley hills, Alexander had hung a number of ancient rugs. Some of them were only fragments. The really old ones were made in mosques or under the direction of Sufis. These rugs, Alexander said, taught him about geometry and order.

They had, he said, "a degree of oneness . . . an inadequate word for something we might call grace or coherence or wholeness."

He was working on an idea that was elusive, difficult, what Huston Smith called "things that cannot be pinned down."

"Since this is a sort of objectionable theory and not liked in contemporary thought, in order to understand it, I had to get very, very empirical," Alexander said. "And somehow demonstrate this, what I claimed to be an objective set of difference of wholeness, would be detected and formed by different observers independent of personal idiosyncrasies and independent of culture. In doing these things, I found the idea that was most useful — well, two things actually, very similar. One of them is that relative amounts of wholeness in a given situation out there, you can access by whether you experience a certain level of wholeness in yourself. Let's say you are talking about great works of art. When you see a thing, a very great work, a sublimely calm thing, you gaze at it, access it. And you say, 'Well, what's the difference between that thing and another thing which is lesser?' The difference is that somehow you say, 'Well, which is a better picture of myself? Of all of me, everything about me, all that I am.' It's an odd question, but the thing that is more whole will be precisely that one about which you say, 'That's a better picture of myself.' When you make a thing, if you are successful, it begins to have attributes that make a picture of the self: myself, yourself, you recognize yourself in it. . . .

"Why is the nature of order connected to the nature of the self? What is the relationship between the two? . . . You gradually have to come to grips with the fact that when you make something, it has the ability to open a little trap door on the essence of things. You can catch a glimpse of that through the order of an object. That something you catch a glimpse of is the place where self and matter are one thing."

As Ann and I sat by the creek, I thought about what it had been like before and after the restoration. Before, many of the same things — water, plants, banks, a tree — had been in place. But it had been a dreary place. Trash, beer cans, plastic bags, bedraggled weeds. People were not drawn to it; no one sat beside it.

Now, the same: water, plants, a bank, a tree. But it was completely different. I looked down at pool of water and the damp brown sand. The creek was waiting, I felt, for the fish to come back. It was part of an order, waiting to be more alive.

I did not feel so isolated there, behind that glass wall. I felt planted on this earth, mirrored in a wholeness or a grace or another inadequate word.

I lay down at home. Almost immediately my mind filled with images of the chemotherapy room at the Cancer Center, the people sitting in lounge chairs hooked up to IVs.

Then something swam into my head. It was a pool of water, deep, and gracious. It arrived out of nowhere. As this pool filled my thoughts, I realized that if I crammed all the space in my mind with anxiety, every nook and cranny, every corner, then there would be no room for that water to flow.

"Grace fills the empty spaces, but it can only enter where there is a void to receive it," Simone Weil said. "And it is grace itself which makes this void."

Grace itself both creates and fills the void. Then I saw that the image of a pool of water that came into my thoughts originated in the pools of water in the creek. The creek had fed my imagination. Having searched for the right words for prayers, this *prayer* did not begin with words, certainly not with rote prayers from a prayer book. It began with water. The order of the creek was speaking to an order in me.

On Monday evening of Valentine's Day, Dr. Wright called. "I'm leaning toward waiting," he said. "Three months. Then we'll do another CT scan."

I asked him if we could do another needle biopsy at another place. He said yes. "Cottage Hospital is good, but you were so miserable the last time."

"Well, yes," I said, "but less miserable than I would be with an open lung."

"We can do that if it's grown in two months," he said.

"What about the lymph nodes?" I asked.

"I think it's calcification. Likely benign."

"If it's not cancer, what is it?"

"I don't know. Some kind of granuloma. Inflamed."

Henri Nouwen said you live either in the house of fear or in the house of love. Henry James said we are either anxious or comatose. The Nouwen was a bit sentimental. The James, a bit cynical. But what they both understood was that the two states are separate, distinct. You are either in one or the other.

I lived in one, and then I lived in the other. I imagined that precious time was being wasted, the cancer was growing. Then, briefly, I lived in another house, in which Dr. Wright and Dr. Mesipam knew what they were doing, and what mattered was the bough of the tree outside my window that seemed to sway whether there was a breeze or not.

I gave a dollar to a man at a freeway exit in his rain poncho who sang out to me, "Be careful driving," and I thanked him and told him I'd take care of myself, doing the best I could. And I felt much less like Lady Bountiful than like this man's companion, in need of his good wishes.

Vincent and I told Dr. Wright we agreed with him — we wanted to wait. A month. Possibly two. He said that was fine. But I did not know how I was going to live through it.

Other people, alerted to this new possibility, went into action. I saw that cancer causes a lot more excitement than an auto-immune disorder. When Dr. Rao talked to me about the PET scan, he held my hand the entire time. I saw later that he was not only comforting me, he was modeling behavior for his two residents, who stood near the door. Dr. Mesipam's quiet nurse was quieter. Dr. Wright answered my e-mails immediately. But one afternoon I called a friend who had just been diagnosed with thyroid cancer — a "mild" form of cancer, her doctors had said.

"I remembered when I terminated analysis," Andra said. "I had thought it would be a huge day, full of insights. It was not the fireworks I thought it would be, but just another day. And I thought yesterday that maybe death is like that. Maybe it's just another day, not such a big deal. My mother watched *Jeopardy* a half hour before she died. And she enjoyed it."

I lay on the window seat looking up at the tree outside, its branches swaying in the imperceptible wind.

For the briefest of seconds, I understood and accepted that death is part of the order of things. It is not separate, distinct, unreal. And then: the bigger we are, the harder it is to die.

I had been made small by being sick, and in that smallness I saw the order of the creek. I saw the man by the freeway, the blind woman in the restaurant, the man in the train station. We are vulnerable, all of us: the creek, the others, and me. It is the order of things to be vulnerable. The disorder is imagining that we are not.

A few days later I couldn't stand waiting any longer.

I asked Vincent: "Would you go back to the Mayo Clinic with me to have another needle biopsy?"

"Yes," he said.

I called Mayo and sent them the PET scan. Dr. Stevens, the neurologist, set up an appointment for a needle biopsy and another one, with the pulmonary division, for a breathing test and a consultation.

We flew into Minneapolis and were driven down the next day in a shuttle in a sweeping snowstorm that rose and fell with the hills between the two cities. We did not want to rent a car this time, figuring in March in Rochester we might not want to go on excursions. We had to save money.

March at Mayo was quite different from October. The two ladies on the scooters and the woman with the cat were nowhere to be seen. In fact, there was almost no one on the street. The streets, as I watched them through the window of the Kahler Inn, looked like frozen iron. Vincent jauntily went out for a walk after we arrived and came back in a matter of minutes, his face red. He put his hands under the blanket on the bed. "Cold," he said.

Staying in the hotel on our floor was a girls' basketball team, and so in the elevators, whenever we went up or down, there was usually some tall girl in sweats, her hair lank and loose and her body in a feverish excitement. Every time I saw one of them, she cheered me up.

The next day, Wednesday, our first appointment was with Dr. Stevens. The receptionist, in Mayo style, told me that he was in the lab, but she would text him to tell him we were early and ask him to come over. I sat in his waiting area, watching a young woman manage to walk from her wheelchair to the reception desk with a smile of triumph on her face.

A nurse led us to an examining room. Dr. Stevens arrived in his customary tweed, blue this time. His brow was furrowed. He washed his hands at the sink and shook hands with both of us. He told me that I would get the schedule at his front desk and then return to see him when I was finished. When I told him that I had tested positive for antiretinal antibodies, he picked up the phone and said, "A lot of that research was done here, so I think I'll call the retinal people." He waited. He pressed down a button and dialed another number. "Hum," he said. "I wonder where they are?" He tried another extension. "All in a meeting?" And then another. He hung up and said, "I wonder if they've gone to the moon.

"Talk to Dr. Leavitt about this," he said, "and if she isn't able to help, talk to me again before you leave." He wished us well, his brow still creased, and I couldn't tell whether the lab was preoccupying him or he was worried about me.

We picked up the schedule at his front desk. The next day, Thursday, I was to have a chest X-ray, a "pulmonary function test," and a blood test.

On Friday I was to report to St. Mary's Hospital for the needle biopsy.

We moved from the Kahler Inn that afternoon to the Kahler Grand, just around the corner. Despite the basketball players, the old Kahler had felt more depressing than in the fall. We needed a change of scene, Vincent said. Our new hotel was pretty spiffy by comparison, not much more expensive, and it had a swimming pool on the top, under a big glass dome, where I could swim, then lie beside it in steamy warm air, looking out on the cold sky.

In a cozy restaurant downstairs with a Dickensian name, Vincent ordered a glass of scotch, and I declined a drink. The waitress gently said, "The bartender has figured out a nonalcoholic drink, a sort of juice thing I call a prom fling." She hesitated. "For those people on meds."

"I'm on meds," I said, "and I'll take one."

On Thursday, during my breathing test, the nurse asked me who I was seeing in pulmonary. Looking at my sheet, I said, "Mr. Holland," registering for the first time that he was a Mister, not a Doctor.

"He is very good," she said. "Excellent."

I Googled Mr. Holland when I returned to the hotel and found that he was a physician's assistant. I felt cheated.

At some point in the early afternoon, I

either became anxious about the needle biopsy or I had a moment of clarity. I called the pulmonary desk and asked them if they could check with the doctors — would a bronchoscopy work as well? They said they would call me back. When they did, they told me, "The needle biopsy is canceled for now. Cart before the horse. They have rescheduled a CT scan for the morning. You can pick up the new schedule at the pulmonary desk."

I was surprised and relieved and also disappointed. I had been gathering my energy for the biopsy, and now, I told myself, it was just going to happen later, and I'd have to gather up my courage again. But for now, it made more sense to talk to pulmonary before the biopsy.

After I picked up my new schedule, I was walking past the Center for the Spirit on my way to the subway to the hotel when I turned around and went back. The etched-glass door slid open. The prayer wall had many pieces of the cream paper on it, slipped in here and there. I stood in front of them and tried to think of writing a prayer for others, but all that came out was "Help me." I pushed it into a slot, then wondered who cleaned the prayers out and whether the person read them. The prayer cleaner. I hoped that person had been one of us, a resident of Oz. I wanted the someone who removed my prayer from its place on the wall to be a person who knew what it was like to be afraid of leaving this world. To know the meaning of the word *befallen*. I wanted the prayer cleaner to have had a spot on his or her lung. To have sat across from a doctor who said, "If she were my wife, I'd take it out." To have heard a radiologist intoning on a tape, "The area appears to be malignant." To have heard a doctor say, "Our radiologist is alarmed." I wondered if Jesus had not only crossed over into the land of suffering, when he took the blind beggar by the hand, but had stayed there. Maybe Jesus was a prayer cleaner.

That night after dinner, on our way back to the hotel, we walked past a small city park. Hundreds of crows were gathered in the trees. They covered every tree, muttering to each other, and occasionally one or two would fly from one tree to another. They must have been trying to keep warm by some combination of gathering and flight. Neither one of us had ever seen so many crows in one place, and we stood watching them even though we were cold. The fear that had been sitting farther out on the fringes of my mind (in a warm restaurant with a friendly waitress) moved into the center. I was just a small thing in a bleak landscape of cold and gray. I stood there while the birds fluttered and cawed, and a few of them moved from tree to tree, and through my coat, the cold seeped in.

In the morning, I took the subway into the main clinic building, then into the lobby of another building that had a strange funeral fountain in it and a pool that people had turned into a wishing well, with coins on the bottom. A vase with flowers only made it worse.

I took the elevator to the second floor where, hanging on the wall, was the beautiful rug with horses dancing across it. The patients waiting were watching the tsunami in Japan on TV, waves flooding into houses, over and over again.

The nurse asked me if I was wearing any metal, and when I assured her I was not, she believed me. I did not have to change into the awful nightie. When I walked into the room with the scan, the technician looked doubtful.

"Any —" he began.

The nurse held up her hand. "She's home free."

"Great," he said. "We'll have you out of here in no time."

It took three minutes.

Vincent was surprised to see me back at the hotel. "Did you do the CT scan?"

"Yes, I think I did," I said.

Our appointment with Mr. Holland was at one o'clock, so we had an early lunch in the hotel, which was directly across the street, and then walked over. I carried my bag with tests, scans, and reports that went with me everywhere like the packs on a horse. And my small black notebook with the lists of questions. In this case, I really had only one.

In the clinic lobby, a man with a long beard and an angry red face crossed and almost stumbled with what looked like a new prosthesis. Two men were sitting at the piano, one playing and the other wearing that open expression that meant he was about to sing. They were both in their late sixties, I guessed, and as I watched them, I saw a family resemblance. They might be brothers. As we passed them on the way to the elevators, I happened to look down and saw that the man playing had only one leg.

I girded myself as we rose in the elevator. A young man dressed in black leather, with light, floating tattoos of birds on his arms, got in on the second floor and moved to the back. I heard a mechanical, fuzzy voice say,

"I think it's floor ten." I turned, and the young man was holding a microphone to his throat to speak.

We sat in the large waiting area for pulmonary, a place I had never been. It was not far from the windows that had the same view as my swimming pool. The sky was the color of steel. It was twenty-two degrees at one o'clock. In California, March meant spring. A jigsaw puzzle sitting on a low table lacked one piece.

I was jumpy. I could not sit still. Vincent sat patiently and methodically working. I was irritated at him: he could work, and I could not.

A nurse called us, from double doors that opened automatically, and led us down a hall where, she said, Mr. Holland would soon join us. An old loden coat hung from a hook on the inside of the door. I felt as if I were entering a cage, a dark cell.

A man in his forties walked in, dark short hair, and a brisk manner. We had a moment of awkwardness where we both stuck our hands out at the same time, and he tried to shake my hand first, missed, and shook Vincent's hand, and then we all sat down. I felt my heart in my throat.

"One thing," he said, looking right at me. "I have looked at all your scans, including the one done this morning, and I am ninety percent sure you do not have cancer."

It was almost imperceptible, the way the living world came back. The room felt suddenly ordinary: a couch, chairs, the high examining table. The silence that had walked beside me since I pulled over to hear Dr. Wright's message was replaced by a soft background hum.

"May I hug you?" I said, and Mr. Holland looked down at his shoes and said yes.

"I am going to lead you through the scans," he said, "but first tell me your story." I started with the blur at the edge of my eye and began to walk through the months: the arterial biopsy, the lumbar puncture, the CT scan in February, the CT scan in May, the CT scan in November. The needle biopsy. The collapsed lung. Mr. Holland interrupted me often. He was clearly waiting, like a cat with a bird in its mouth.

Finally he said, "Anyone mention *sarcoidosis* to you?"

A word. Sarcoidosis. I told him that Dr. Wright had mentioned it early on, as a possibility, and the rheumatoid specialist at UCLA had wondered about it, but nothing had come of it. I told him I had read about neuro-sarcoidosis, on the Mayo Web site, and had mentioned it to a fellow in ophthalmology, who had dismissed it. I realized, as I talked to him, that it had been floating in the air, without traction, for at least a year.

I said, "My mother had it."

"Really!" he said. "When was she diagnosed? Where was it found? How did it manifest?"

"I was a teenager. My mother had a spot on her lung. They thought it was cancer. My father took her to Houston." I remembered them packing.

"Ah," he said. "Let me show you the scans."

He centered himself in front of the screen at his desk and walked us through each one.

"Slices of the body," he said, and brought up a grainy image of something that looked like a creature from *Alien,* with sockets for eyes and a dome with cavities in it. I made out a band of ribs around two spaces with pieces of things in them, like wisps of string and one weird spiral-shaped thing. Upper left. My eyes fixed on it.

"We're looking down from the head to the toes, in one-millimeter slices," Mr. Holland said, typing at the keyboard. "This is the left side. Here's the spot in February. And now in May." He turned toward me. "Same size, right?"

"Right," I said.

"And now in November," he said, bringing up the image. The spiral was now a largish blob.

I shrank from it.

"It's grown," he said.

"Yikes," I said, trying to sound nonchalant.

"Yep," he said, "but not to get concerned, because here we have today's scan."

On the screen was the same image, the same lung, but the blob had become a small oblong.

"It's smaller," Mr. Holland said, turning back toward me. "Cancer doesn't get smaller." Then he continued, "I am ninety-nine percent sure. I read scans all day. I canceled the biopsy when I saw your scans. Even before I saw today's scan."

He turned back to the screen, then hesitated and said, "By the way, at Mayo, we never do PET scans unless we have a confirmed case of cancer. To see if it's metastasized. To see if the tumors have grown."

"Never?"

"Never. We do not use PET scans as a diagnostic tool."

I went blank for a moment. Then a rage that I first misinterpreted as confusion filled my brain, up to the sockets, right up to the corpus callosum. The Mayo Clinic, surely an authoritative place that a doctor might consult, doesn't use PET scans to diagnose disease.

Mr. Holland left us, and briefly, a doctor came in and confirmed what Mr. Holland had said.

He and Mr. Holland ordered a broncho-scopy, explaining that they would look in the lymph nodes for noncaseating granulo-mas, the standard test for "sarcoid," as well as "sweep" the lung for cells and get as close to the lesion, or whatever it was, as they could. He gave me a brochure with a pale pink and lavender cover with "Sarcoidosis" written on it. I keep it now as if it were holy scripture.

We had spent a total of forty-five minutes with Mr. Holland and another twenty minutes with the doctor. We walked out of the examining room area through the double doors. As we passed through the hall, I saw Mr. Holland sitting at a computer screen with another doctor looking over his shoulder.

"Thank God," Vincent said, as we walked out the double doors, "we came to this place."

It must have been about four in the

afternoon. They had talked to us as if we were their only patient. I walked across the waiting area toward the floor-to-ceiling windows.

I stood there in the sunlight looking out at the bluffs. A light snow was falling. I called Dr. Mesipam and left a message on his machine. I told him that Mayo had all but ruled out lung cancer. That they thought I had something called sarcoidosis. And what they said about PET scans. How right he had been.

I haven't yet forgotten how I felt that weekend, when I was recalled to life. By the hard work and grace of Mr. Holland, not a doctor, not a priest. For twenty-five years, he had contemplated and become expert at scans. Vincent and I rejoiced, as far as one can in Rochester in March: we feasted at different restaurants for breakfast, lunch, and dinner. We followed the crowds in the subways and the over-the-street walkways to the stadium where our girls played in a basketball tournament. We walked, very briefly, along the icy river. I did not care what we did. The life around me was not mine, not yet. I might never regain the oblivious, but I could walk close to the healthy people near me, and rather than hate them, as I had in the train station in Los Angeles, I could love what they were, living bodies, enfolded, like me, in the world.

On Monday morning a Mayo nurse called me to say they could do the bronchoscopy earlier. I would not have to fast as long.

Back in the pulmonary section, I sat in a lounge chair, and Vincent sat beside me. A nurse stayed with us the whole time. A bronchoscopy is done by sending a flexible tube through the throat and windpipe, into the lungs. It has on it a tiny viewing device. The doctors would also take tissue samples with the same apparatus. Two people came in with a little cart to put in the IV line. Two people, Vincent noted, are more efficient than one, because one is unwrapping the needle while the other is talking and then inserting the needle. Then they were gone.

The nurse said, "They are washing down the room now and drying it. Then you. Very soon. Ready?"

She covered me with two warm blankets and wheeled the chair down the hall. I didn't have to get up. She would be beside me, she said, the whole time. I was to signal with my hand if I was uncomfortable at any time.

260

We entered a dim room where I saw a male doctor and a female doctor. He shook my hand, introduced himself, introduced the woman, a resident, and then they both gloved up. They put a light gauze over my eyes and sprayed what tasted like cough syrup down my throat. They started Versed, the erase-the-memory drug, and Ativan, the I-don't-care drug. I was aware, at some point, of the male doctor saying, "A lot of calcification in there," and I signaled the nurse. They gave me more Ativan. And then they were pulling tubes out of my throat, and we were finished, and the nurse was pushing the chair down the hall to the other room.

She tucked me into a wheelchair. She said to me and to Vincent that she was sorry I had to be in the wheelchair. She asked Vincent where we were parked, and he said we were at the Kahler Grand across the street, and she said, "Oh, just take the chair to your room and leave it somewhere over there, and we'll come get it."

Suddenly we were in the elevator. I felt a mix of relief and self-consciousness: I was in a public place in a wheelchair. We came out of the elevator, and Vincent was wheeling me up the ramp to the street, when I saw a kid in a wheelchair to my left, and we

261

came up beside her. Before this moment I had often looked at people in wheelchairs with a slightly condescending sympathy. Never having figured out what to say, I had often nodded or said hello and then looked away. They were in another country, a place I would never be. And I had always received in return a thank-you-but-no-thank-you look in reply. But this time, as we pulled alongside her, I said, "Hi." And she looked at me with a full open smile, as if we were companions. On the road together.

CHAPTER 17

The bronchoscopy found noncaseating granulomas in my lymph nodes, the definitive test for sarcoidosis. My blood tests found heightened calcium levels, another sign. Mr. Holland did not make a final judgment until after all the cultures of the tissues they had taken inside my lungs had come back negative for everything else. He called me with the news. Indeed, as he had suspected, from the pattern of the scars on the scans, from the lesion that grew and shrank, from the granuloma in my lymph nodes, I had sarcoidosis.

Sarcoidosis was discovered and named in 1899, when the Norwegian dermatologist Caesar Boeck found skin nodules characterized by "compact, sharply defined foci of epithelioid cells with large pale nuclei and also a few giant cells." Thinking this resembled sarcoma, he called the condition "multiple benign sarcoid of the skin."

Sarcoid's marker is microscopic clumps of inflammatory cells, granulomas (found in my lymph nodes), that clump together and leave deep, grainy scars. Think of them, one specialist said, as a football huddle around the elusive cause.

Sarcoid can affect almost any organ in the body. "An enigmatic multisystem disease," said *The New England Journal of Medicine*. When too many of these clumps form in an organ, they can virtually destroy it.

Among autoimmune disorders, it is considered rare, but some specialists think it's far more common than the medical world imagines because it often has no symptoms. One doctor told me that if he took cuts across my body every millimeter, he would find granulomas in every organ.

Researchers think that something in the environment may cause sarcoid. It may be bacteria. Pine smoke or pine resin was a suspect: hence the doctors' interest in the fire I was lighting when I first saw the blur. Mold. Whatever the cause, it is found all over the world, everywhere and in every place.

Those of us who have sarcoid continue to fight its cause with our immune systems, a ghost in our bodies. I, obviously, because of my mother, have a genetic predisposition to it.

Sarcoid can kill. The lungs stiffen, the heart is scarred, the kidneys fail. The entries on sarcoid support group sites are full of pain and sorrow: sarcoid in the throat, in the esophagus, in the lungs. His breathing gets harder and harder, one man wrote, "Please help me keep the will to live."

Because the disease affects so many different parts of the body, a patient can end up with lots of doctors. I have, as of this writing, seven. All of us have a lung specialist, as sarcoid always affects the lungs. It often affects the eyes and kidneys. I am lucky to have such excellent medical insurance, to be able to travel to find the right doctor. To have had the support of my local doctors to persist. (One of my doctors, searching for just the right word to describe me, said, "Oh, Ms. Gallagher, you have been — you have been — a most thorough patient!" I burst out laughing.)

Having a diagnosis changed everything. The long loop in which I had spent my nights — What could I have? Am I on the wrong drugs? What if I have something that requires other drugs? And what if I have lung cancer? What if it was cancer all along that caused this? — that loop was gone.

It changed my doctors' attitudes. I found them to be more focused and, I saw later, less anxious. They knew what they were dealing with. It had a name.

When I was a child, a friend and I played a game: Fortunately and Unfortunately.

"Fortunately," Fred would say, "Pete escaped the shark by climbing into a boat. Unfortunately, the boat had a hole in it."

"Fortunately," I would reply, "a man plugged it up. Unfortunately, the shark bit another hole in the boat."

Fortunately, I had a diagnosis. Unfortunately, very few doctors know very much about sarcoidosis, and almost none of them are on the West Coast. It is not uncommon for a definitive diagnosis of sarcoid to take as long as mine did. (In a comic, "Brief History of Sarcoidosis," posted on a sarcoidosis support site, a fellow patient wrote, "1958: Scientists and doctors from all over the world meet at Brompton Hospital in London for the first ever conference about Sarcoidosis. Since nobody knows anything about the disorder, they shortly retire to brandy and cigars.")

My visual field in the right eye fluctuated again last summer; my hearing in the right ear diminished. Dr. Wright, my lung doctor here, urged me to consult Dr. Robert Baughman, a sarcoid specialist in Cincinnati.

I reminded Dr. Wright that I had been to Mayo. I did not need another specialist. He said, "We still don't have anyone leading our team. This man has done the most research on sarcoid."

Vincent and I had very little expectation when we flew into Cincinnati in early December.

The clinics were almost empty; the temperature outside just above freezing. We sat in yet another examining room. Dr. Baughman walked in, tall and lean, his dark hair cut in a bowl, like a monk. He introduced himself as Bob. Then he said, "You are my last patient of the day. We can take as long as you want. Please tell me your story."

I did. I told him the whole story from beginning to end. He listened. Every now and then he asked a question: "How long have you had uveitis? Did they do an MRI when you were first diagnosed?"

He looked at my tests and scans, and finally he smiled and said, "I think that indeed you do have sarcoidosis," with a brief, wry nod to how long it had taken, how far we had traveled. He suggested that

I gradually switch from methotrexate and prednisone to Remicade, an "anti-TNF inhibitor," borrowed from oncology, to tamp down my immune response.

"It's because," he said, "I am pretty sure that you have neuro-sarcoid." And after that I have very little memory of what he said because my mind went back almost two years, to Dr. J. The examining room, the snap in his voice: *You are looking things up on the Internet.* I had stopped researching neuro-sarcoid after that. I had lost faith in myself.

"I am aggressive about sarcoid," Dr. Baughman said, in his modest office in the late afternoon. "Some doctors are not. I think it's important to use serious drugs against neuro-sarcoid because of the scars the granulomas can leave. Scarring," he said carefully, "can't be fixed." He hesitated. "I would like to make sure that that nerve remains the same or improves. I am an optimist. I think it can improve." He watched me carefully.

On a Web site he showed me a memory test he wanted me to take, and on the BBC Web site a reaction time test involving sheep crossing a meadow, which he almost failed. ("I always get a bad score," he said calmly.) After two and half hours, he said, "I imagine you are tired."

"I am," I said. "And I am grateful."

I took a second to gather my courage and then said, "How do I follow up with you? Is there a chance I might be your patient?"

He fiddled in his jacket pocket and pulled out a business card. "I will send a report to your doctors in California. I would like to see you again in six months. My e-mail is here," he pointed to it. "I will always answer you within twenty-four hours."

He walked us out through the empty corridors until we were oriented, then shook our hands.

"Don't forget to see the Turners at the Taft Museum," he said in parting. "They're very nice."

We walked back to our hotel, a few blocks away, in the cold and the fading light. Vincent said he was going to the bar, and I said I was going to the gym. I worked out slowly, letting my body move and flex.

A young woman who had all the abs and biceps you would ever need came in and grinned. "You look happy," she said.

"I am," I said. "I am in good hands."

Dr. Baughman's attitude and skill and open heart made me more forgiving of the other doctors, even Dr. J. I was in good hands, and so I could afford to be generous. I thought about what doctors were up against: they had one foot in Oz and one in the land of the well, they made a constant effort to get it right, and they paid a price for getting it wrong.

I am and I am not who I was. I have lost part of my vision, part of my hearing, and part of my faith.

When I shop in grocery stores with their narrow aisles, fast-moving mothers and children and carts, I am almost always surprised by someone coming up on the right. I can neither see nor hear them. That chunk of periphery I took for granted that announces a body somewhere on the edge of things is gone. That piece of auditory nerve that picks up the sound of a footfall or the creak of a cart in the distance? That too is gone.

These deaths, if you will, announce the ones sure to come, the diminution of my sentries: hearing, sight.

I would give quite a lot to have my "old" body back, the one that hefted suitcases and traveled here and there and was oblivious. I would give quite a lot not to have to think about drugs and side effects and what happens when you "tamp" down the immune system and open yourself up to shingles,

TB, pneumonia, lymphoma, and melanoma. I would give a lot not to spend so much of my time in doctors' offices, not to read old *National Geographics,* not to know the names of the receptionists and how the bad divorce is going and how the taxi driver in Los Angeles wishes to see his family in Armenia more often.

"Please bring all of your records," Dr. Baughman's office had told me. "But we understand that you are a prepared patient." I would rather not be "a prepared patient." I would rather not have to track down the latest MRI, the latest CT scan, the blood work, the X-ray, the list of medicines. I know now to keep that list on my body at all times so that I don't have to write down all of them, including "over the counter," once again, on the form that no one, except the Mayo Clinic and Dr. Baughman, seems to read. I know now to ask for a copy of one doctor's report to another and read it through because it will always contain at least one error, which I will then have to correct.

I would rather not know that the mail order pharmacy must be checked for inject-able methotrexate, because it is likely that they don't have it, and therefore my local pharmacist, who always has it, will have to

271

receive from my medical insurance a "one-time override." I would rather not know how to inject methotrexate.

But the new drugs are effective. I am glad to live at a time when they are available. And this is what is real now.

Some months ago I was sitting on a staircase outside my retinologist's office because his waiting room had so many patients in it, there was no place to sit. A tall woman with dark hair joined me there, and after a while we traded stories. I was no longer aloof from other patients, no longer pretending this was a way station. She told me finally about the effort it took to hide her increasing blindness from her employer and colleagues so she could keep her job.

My own "challenges" are nothing, of course, compared to hers and to others': shunts for chemotherapy, bone marrow transplants, isolation wards, joint pain from lupus, gradual disintegration caused by MS. The slow deterioration from age.

We pretend to ourselves that it won't happen to us. *About suffering, they were never wrong . . .* I won't get sick; I will not die. William Saroyan is quoted as saying on his deathbed: "Everybody has got to die, but I have always believed there would be an exception in my case." I saw an old woman crossing the street, and what traveled through my mind was, *My skin won't sag that much, my knees will not buckle.*

When Jodie looked up at me, her hands full of Frank's ashes, I looked away.

And so we sit here: the woman hiding her blindness, the child in the wheelchair at the Mayo Clinic, Jodie in her bedroom that day, and me — on one side of the glass wall.

What I want from the church, or any faith community, I see now, is a look between human beings that says we are knitted together, standing in a circle, holding each other up, waiting for the next ax to fall, rather than persons following a crowned Jesus, believing in an oppressive creed and tinny, false hope. That "religion" is about wanting the thing to last forever and make the pain go away. The reality is, instead, more about Jesus kneeling in the dust making a paste of spit and dirt. The reality is much more raw.

He lived in the country of the sick and forsaken. He left a map of it, his own *derrotero.* (This smaller, individual map, we forget, is the basis of the larger one.) Jesus knew the streets and the houses. The way it feels to be afraid, hurt, unattended, ignored, tortured. To be vulnerable. Jesus took this *information* back to the order at the heart of the universe.

It is a kind of desecration that we made of this man, a crown, a king, a Lord. Jesus is about as far away from a king as a person can be.

And if we are to take Jesus as an indication of what god's nature is like — not because Jesus is god's only son, but because Jesus seemed to have committed himself to following out to the end what he thought god was — god ends up here with the sick and the dying, too. A voluntary citizen of Oz.

And where, you may very well ask, does that get us? I seem not to be able to answer the question. It appears to be in the nature of this particular god to have been the opposite of the God as King celebrated in Christian churches. God is not the Father Almighty.

That's the faith I lost. I lost a faith I had been about to lose for years, a faith based on an empire's pleasure and not on a young man's compassion. I lost what faith I had in the map based on conquest and not on discovery.

When I looked at the girl at Mayo and she looked back, I had the uncanny sense that there was a third person there. He was there because she was there. And I was there. We were willing to be there, together, on the road, just that, nothing more. A very fragile line connected us, as fragile as the water in the creek. The life in her smile helped get me through my recovery. We were parts of the order at the heart of things. And so whoever this man was, who lived and died and then lived again, was there, too. Jesus, as Mark Benson said of his partner, Philip, is no longer literal, not here, not visible, but not absent, not without influence, not dead.

The resurrection, when looked at this way, is not a magic act but the revelation of what stays alive and what dies. Vulnerability and its close cousin, love, stay alive. The rest? Clanging cymbals. Sounding brass.

And in the end, as you know, so you are known. In the end, you will be greeted as a friend and not a stranger.

Jesus was on his way to Jerusalem when he came across the blind man sitting in the road. He took him by the hand and walked with him out of the village. There he mixed together dust and dirt. He placed this paste over the sightless eyes. Here is what we might do for each other, those of us in Oz, those outside it. He knelt in the dust not to "fix" the blindness but to be there inside the suffering. This doesn't mean entering into the suffering for suffering's sake (the mistake made by hair shirts and kneeling on cold stone), or a boundaryless, oozy sharing, but instead a way to hold it, to sit with it, to accept our mutual vulnerability. Not to solve it. Not to give advice.

Jodie once described this by cupping her hands together as if she were holding a tiny bird. To be willing to feel what comes our way from the distant and very close land of pain. The terror, the pain, the catastrophe that is no one's fault. This gesture of acceptance is the most helpful thing because it recognizes the person suffering not as a stranger but as a friend, a fellow sufferer. Because, of course, you will be next.

One spring day in New York, in my former life, I came out of the subway on the same street as I usually did to get to MOMA, and rather than cross the street and turn left, I turned right, away from the museum, and toward Fifth Avenue. On the avenue I turned right again, to walk south. Just ahead of me, on the corner of East 50th, was a huge Gothic church. St. Patrick's Cathedral, star of movies and song, and never without people. Never without someone praying or lighting a candle or just walking around, a feeling inside its stone walls of being at the heart of something old, and you could use all the words that people mouth when trying to pass a political correctness test — *diverse, multigenerational, color-blind* — and not get at what I felt every time I walked in, which was *Wow, the whole city is here.*

St. Patrick's had a very long line of people waiting along one side. I counted at least three hundred bodies. At the head of the line was a sign: ashes. I passed them and made my way a couple of blocks east to St. Bartholomew's Episcopal Church, where the noon service for Ash Wednesday had just begun.

When I entered the huge bronze doors to St. Bart's, far up the long, long aisle, I could see a young blond priest. She said, "Almighty God, you have created us out of the dust of the earth . . ."

Under the huge Byzantine dome of the church, the dark suits of midtown Manhattan, accountants and lawyers and Merrill Lynch brokers — hundreds of men and women — were kneeling. I crept up the aisle and knelt down with the rest of them.

Next in the service was the imposition of ashes, and I joined the others, walked up to the altar, and waited. A priest told me I was dust and to dust I would return and placed black soot on my forehead. Once it was done, I walked back to the pew, as I have done many times in my life on Ash Wednesdays past, and sat down. The rest of the service commenced: we considered our sins, which, in the new prayer book of the Episcopal Church, include things like "waste and pollution of creation," and "prejudice and contempt toward those who differ from us," and "our intemperate love of worldly goods and comforts and our dishonesty in daily life and work." We took a brief and austere communion. Then we got up and walked back out toward the world. Only then, and only because I looked around at my fellow sinners, did it occur to me that we all had black marks on our foreheads. And then, that we were all in a city where you did not, most of the time, enjoy the anonymity of a car. Always before, on Ash Wednesday, with that unmistakable mark on my face, I'd slunk quickly back to the car and driven home. I'm a writer, I work at home, so the decision about whether to remove the smudge is a pretty low-level one.

But I was in New York, my face on public display. Damn, I thought. Was this the time to take a taxi? I couldn't tell if anyone else cared at all. Then what came to my mind very clearly was the memory of a man I had passed on the sidewalk the day before. He

278

was selling scarves and socks and batteries
— those things for sale in sidewalk stands
all over New York — but at that moment he
was not selling; he was on his knees on a
little piece of carpet, crammed into a little
spot near his table, right up against the legs,
his left foot nearly in the street. As I slowed
down, he folded himself over and placed his
forehead on the concrete, facing east,
toward Mecca. He was praying. He was
praying in New York. *And I too am praying,* I
thought, as I walked out into the cool spring
air, where the pink tulips were budding on
the dividers on Park Avenue. I too was praying in New York. I was praying to end my
waste and pollution, my prejudice and
contempt, my intemperate love of comfort
and worldly goods.

I walked down Park Avenue, away from
the subway. I don't know what made me
turn left instead of right. Soon I was walking past a copy shop, a small place that
probably serviced both the midtown offices
around it and also Grand Central Station.
A young woman was standing practically in
the window, opening a copy machine's lid,
a piece of paper in her hand. Just as I
passed, she looked up, and I saw there, on
her forehead, a dark, unmistakable smudge.
I felt a jolt of pleasure. She looked up just

as I passed, and we exchanged a look of odd recognition: *Oh, you . . . too?* I didn't break stride, I was in New York after all. But it dawned on me within half a block that there would be others — and then I knew why I had decided to walk rather than scoot home on the subway.

I crossed through Grand Central Station, parting the sea of people under the stars of its dome, and a man carrying a briefcase was smudged; also a woman with a seeing-eye dog. I passed the Algonquin Hotel on West 44th Street, and the doorman, in his heavy green coat, turned, and there on his forehead was a blur of ash. When I was closer to home, in the Village, I took a saunter down Bleecker Street and passed August, a hip restaurant with dark booths and a beautiful glassed-in garden room. At a table near the window sat a woman in fur reading the menu, and right on her fore-head, when she turned to look out at the street, was a dark smear.

They were such different people: the young woman at the copier, the doorman at the Algonquin, the woman in fur having lunch. Who knows what drew them to that particular faith on that particular day? I did not wash my face when I got home. I wanted to be identified as part of this collective noun, like an exaltation of larks or a covey of geese, a scattering of followers. Followers, not believers. Marked by dust. The dust that Jesus used to mix with saliva to make a paste. The dust to which we will all return.

I think of them now, and their untold stories, their unread maps.

The doctors can measure the changes in my sight and my hearing, but only I can measure the part of my faith I lost.

You will find me in church on Sundays, but not in the pew. Instead, I sit with a few others in a small chapel to the side of the main sanctuary in a twenty-minute meditation between services. A tiny heater buzzes on the floor.

Through the walls I can hear the choir practicing various familiar hymns.

It is the right metaphor for me: I hear them but only through the walls. I am in a different but related room.

I am glad to be freed from saying words that have ceased to be mine. The loss of old words has left space for new ones, here, written down. I went into exile and came out with something else; I am reimagining the nature of faith or, at least, of my faith. As are so many others.

■ ■ ■ ■

And while you will not find me in a regular church service on Sunday, I have regard, more than regard, for the effort made there over the centuries to describe and come to terms with our human condition, to find a moral bearing in the midst of death and suffering. A weight gathered up, prayers sent into the air, institutional continuation. A place for me to sit in silence. And a place that captures the old words, the foundational stories. I went to an Easter Vigil recently, just to sit in the dark with the others, and listened to the words from the temple priest and poet Ezekiel: "Create in me a clean heart, O Lord."

I miss the company on a Sunday, the unexpected jostle, the tears that come unexpectedly, the stranger next to me when I take communion. The reminder of people in need. I take communion on Thursdays when I can, at noon, with the base community. I need the bread and wine.

I now take a Sabbath, borrowed (very loosely) from Judaism. On Saturday I put away the Internet. I don't watch TV. I do not work. Other than that, I do what I want. I don't follow the old road of Christian suffering for the sake of suffering, so I don't set for myself more things not to do. Sometimes I sit in the backyard with Junior the cat. Sometimes I cook. Sometimes I nap.

Four times a week I meditate. At Trinity, twice a week, the rest at home. I have always disliked the idea of meditation. It was either "some weird thing out of India" that I heard about in my adolescence or some weird thing people talked about, a few times too often, in California.

But a friend I respect had taken me to Quaker meetings in New York to sit in the long silence that's at the core of that faith, and when I emerged from an hour of silence, the leaves on the trees outside were sharper. A white-haired man had stood up at the end and said, "I have been thinking we are a body waiting for truth."

What finally got me to start meditating regularly was not only Jodie's question about where I was putting my mind, but a practitioner of acupuncture who has her own immune disorder. A woman of intelligence and experience, she told me that meditation creates "another matrix" besides the fretful mind worrying about illness.

The image of a *matrix,* a nonspiritual word, appealed to me. As did her mind, and her own suffering. And so I kept dragging myself to the meditation sessions at Trinity. They were agonizing eternities. Then one week I went as a thirsty woman to water. And very briefly, in the midst of the half hour, I had a moment where I felt the nearness of something, *a presence.*

"Imagine God, or the presence, or what you want to call it," said a young man who teaches meditation, "just about six inches from your nose."

"Imagine," he said the next week, "that you are very good at this."

The next night, as I lay in bed fretting, I reminded myself, as I have done before without success, that what I was thinking *had not happened yet.* And in second or two, I was back in the present — in a warm bed. I was in the infinite, raw present — and the present's "information."

When Jodie asked me, on the beach in December 2009, what I would do if I went blind, and I said that I would not know how to live, I see now — *see* now — that what was real then would not be what would be real should I go blind. I could imagine, then on that beach, that if I went blind, I would not be able to live. But if it happened, if it happened . . . it would have its own reality, its own *information.* The truth is, I would not know until I got there.

The meditation I am learning comes from the East. The Jesus I follow comes from Christianity but, I hope, from the originator of that faith, before it was co-opted. The cup I drink from is like one at the Metropolitan Museum of Art in New York — a *kernos,* a vase for "multiple offerings" made during the Cycladic culture two thousand years before the birth of Jesus.

Following Jesus was meant to be an ongoing movement, not a creed, not a wall of set-in-stone words. A place where practices, like prayer, like meditation, were taught; where stories and memories, largely about vulnerability and suffering, were collected and shared. The body's pain and suffering were meant to be part of this whole: I don't think Jesus had in mind a place where you had to tolerate the *empty predictability of a service* and stand upright at the coffee hour if you had been diagnosed with lymphoma or sarcoidosis or lung cancer. He was, at the heart of his ministry, a healer.

And the stories of his followers were meant to be taken seriously, to become part of the ongoing larger Story. A river of stories, joining the sea. The living stories of a faith's followers are what keep it alive.

I have more regard for how each of us finds a way; the man in scrubs playing the

Moonlight Sonata at the Mayo Clinic, the girl in the wheelchair, the boy with no hair running in the wind, each of us feeling our way in the dark. "The infinite value of one human being," a friend said, "isn't that what it's all about?"

This land of illness, behind the wall, is much larger than I thought, and through its lens, the world we all live in, what we call the natural world, becomes more precious. I said I would give quite a lot to have my old body back, but yesterday I *saw* the evening light falling on the old oak trees in our park, their bark like the skins of elephants. This world is so beautiful, and not only can I still see it, I no longer pass through it quite the same way I did before. I, at least sometimes, am in it, in its beauty, in its enchantment, in its divine life. I would not trade this *information* for more speaking engagements or for all the riches (or most of them) in the world. Would I trade it for the old oblivious-ness? Maybe so. Maybe not.

In early December last year, I went for a regular visit to Dr. Rao, in the church season of Advent, a time of waiting. My vi-sion was not as good as last time, probably due to the cataracts forming in the left eye because of the steroids. The visual field was better.

I sat in the room by myself, and then very quietly, almost without a sound, Dr. Rao opened the door and came in. I felt stilled. The room was stilled. It became in those moments, like the chapel in which I sit, a place that has been filled with concentrated grace. Coherence. Or some other word.

Dr. Rao was slower. He greeted me quietly. He shook my hand. Rather than talk to me at all, he simply arranged his stool to look at my dilated eyes. I said nothing.

Dr. Nazari, his new fellow, from Iran, slipped into the room. He stood in the corner and watched his teacher.

Dr. Rao looked at my eyes with so much concentration I could barely breathe. I thought about how many eyes he had looked at over the course of a lifetime. So many different arrangements of sight. Light. Color. These things that allow us to see. To see the world. To see the sycamore trees, the butterfly, Vincent's face. He switched to the other eye. With the same concentration. I felt an immense gratitude to this man who has spent his life looking at eyes and that he was still in the room looking at mine.

Dr. Nazari had not moved.

Then Dr. Rao took from his white jacket

pocket the magnifying glass that all ophthal-
mologists carry and slowly, with the same
concentration, brought it to his eye to look
at the back of my eye. He looked at the
other eye. He sat back. He scooted his stool
over to the counter and made notes on the
drawing of my eye for that day.

He turned when he was finished, moved
his stool back so that he was sitting beside
me, and said, "From an ophthalmological
point of view, it all looks calm. No uveitis.
The nerve is not inflamed but farther back"
— he gestured with his hand — "farther
back. It must be."

"So you think it's neuro-sarcoid," I said.

"Oh yes, neuro-sarcoid," he replied softly.
"The visual field has improved." He
smiled, gently. He looked carefully at me.
Did I understand that? his expression said.

"Yes," I said. "I am so glad."

Dr. Nazari, in the corner, smiled.

Dr. Rao cleared up his thoughts and told
Dr. Nazari to send a note to Dr. Baughman, the sarcoid specialist. Then he was out
the door.

A few nights later I lay in bed. Unbidden,
two words came to me: "You are . . ." Other
words piled up behind them: *the kingdom?
the power?* And then they were indistinct. I

was trying to remember something; was it a prayer or a hymn? And then I saw a pond, a small piece of water that was, I understood, me or what I might call the words I have not used yet here, my soul. And on its edge, a border, a ragged line. Then another body of water, much larger, deep, stretching out to a horizon I could not see. As if two pieces of a jigsaw were about to be fitted together. "You are," I said. And then, again, "You are."

ACKNOWLEDGMENTS

Acknowledgments have a deeper meaning and feel inadequate when people have saved your life. I hope that all of those named here know that this is the current that lies under the thanks.

I thank my editor, Jane Garrett, for years of dedication, thoughtful ideas, strength, compassion, and courage, and Leslie Levine, for shepherding the manuscript through its final stages. I am deeply grateful to Chip Kidd for the cover of the original publisher's edition. Thank you to Janet Biehl for her excellent copyediting and to Victoria Pearson for overseeing production editorial.

Jodie Ireland, Bill Powers, and Gary Hall gave me ideas about the manuscript's strengths and weaknesses. This would not be a book without the three of you.

My agent, Philippa Brophy, read the manuscript and insisted on the revisions that turned out to be essential. Thank you.

And thank you Julia Kardon, for your time and intelligence.

The Patagonia environmental team — Lisa Pike-Sheehy, Lisa Myers, Hans Cole, and Ron Hunter — carried more of my workload than they told me. Thank you.

I am grateful to Patagonia's Susan Henderson for stubbornly working through the medical insurance maze.

I thank these excellent teachers: Kristi Cooper White, Diane Barrickman, Amy Havens.

I thank Malinda Chouinard for all that she did but especially for Cincinnati.

I thank my friends for the extra hours of driving, tending, cooking, accompanying to doctors' appointments, and what we call "support" that turns out to be sacrifice: Ellin Barret, Marie Schoeff, Ann Jaqua, Jodie Ireland, Elizabeth Garnsey, Cynthia Gorney, Terry Roof, and Art Stevens.

For the steadfastness from afar that kept me going: Martha Sherrill, Andra Lichtenstein, Harriet Barlow, Alice Gordon, Barbara Brown Taylor, Debbie Sears, and John Lindner.

For the sweetness and love: Jennifer, Rick, Carissa, and Dwight and Claire Chouinard and Matt Stoecker.

I thank Josh Stern and Sarah Key for

always looking after me. And I am grateful for Alison and Jim Stern and for John Stern, in memory.

I thank my parish priest, Mark Asman, for all that he puts up with; for his deep, abiding faith; and for his immediate help in any emergency.

This book is partially dedicated to Dr. Babji Mesipam, but here I want to thank him particularly. Without the support of at least one doctor, a patient cannot persist. Dr. Mesipam was that doctor for me. I am grateful to Robert Wright for his own persistence. Drs. Bevra Hahn and Les Dorfman, human and humane specialists, and Dr. Hossein Nazari, for his skill and compassion. Drs. Laura Koth and Jeffrey Gelfand, at UCSF for spirit and dedication. Dr. Gelfand is the only doctor I have seen come out to the waiting room to find and shepherd his patients. Thank you, Dr. Jennifer Derebery, for determination and brilliance. I am grateful to Dr. Randy Howard for analysis and research, freely given. I thank Dr. Marc Lowe for his early identification and quick response. I am very grateful to Dianna Garner and also Lily Hopkins. I am thankful for Sara Person-Isaacs and Monica Nungaray at Dr. Mesipam's office. I thank Steve Cooley and Ann Marie Granaroli at Sansum Pharmacy.

Thank you, Jason Handler and Celia Dermont, healers. Thank you, Dr. Dawn George, always.

I am deeply grateful to Robert Baughman for time, expertise, compassion, and dedication.

And I am grateful to Dr. Karl Golnik for his experience, skill, and follow-up.

I thank the Mayo Clinic, Roberta Allan, and Tom Brokaw.

Thank you Nan and Craig and Luke. Without you . . .

And finally I thank Vincent, my heart. You showed me what the vow looks like.

— *Nora Gallagher,*
Santa Barbara, Summer 2012

ABOUT THE AUTHOR

Nora Gallagher is the author of *Changing Light, Things Seen and Unseen: A Year Lived in Faith,* and *Practicing Resurrection: A Memoir of Work, Doubt, Discernment, and Moments of Grace.* Her essays, book reviews, and journalism have appeared in *The New York Times Magazine, The Washington Post, DoubleTake,* and *Mother Jones,* among other publications. She is also the editor of the award-winning *Notes from the Field,* a collection of literary essays about the outdoors.